# TALKING POINTS IN DERMATOLOGY – III

Other titles in the *New Clinical Applications* Series:

**Dermatology** (Series Editor Dr J. L. Verbov)
*Dermatological Surgery*
*Superficial Fungal Infections*
*Talking Points in Dermatology – I*
*Treatment in Dermatology*
*Current Concepts in Contact Dermatitis*
*Talking Points in Dermatology – II*
*Tumours, Lymphomas and Selected Paraproteinaemias*
*Relationships in Dermatology*

**Cardiology** (Series Editor Dr D. Longmore)
*Cardiology Screening*

**Rheumatology** (Series Editors Dr J. J. Calabro and Dr W. Carson Dick)
*Ankylosing Spondylitis*
*Infections and Arthritis*

**Nephrology** (Series Editor Dr G. R. D. Catto)
*Continuous Ambulatory Peritoneal Dialysis*
*Management of Renal Hypertension*
*Chronic Renal Failure*
*Calculus Disease*
*Pregnancy and Renal Disorders*
*Multisystem Diseases*
*Glomerulonephritis I*
*Glomerulonephritis II*

NEW
CLINICAL
APPLICATIONS
**DERMATOLOGY**

# TALKING POINTS IN DERMATOLOGY – III

Editor

JULIAN L. VERBOV
JP, MD, FRCP, FIBiol

Consultant Dermatologist
Royal Liverpool Hospital,
Liverpool, UK

**KLUWER ACADEMIC PUBLISHERS**
DORDRECHT / BOSTON / LONDON

**Distributors**

*for the United States and Canada*: Kluwer Academic Publishers, PO Box 358, Accord Station, Hingham, MA 02018–0358, USA
*for all other countries*: Kluwer Academic Publishers Group, Distribution Center, PO Box 322, 330 AH Dordrecht, The Netherlands

**British Library Cataloguing in Publication Data**

Talking points in dermatology. – III
1. Medicine. Dermatology
I. Verbov, Julian II. Series
616.5

ISBN-13: 978-94-010-7687-6 e-ISBN-13: 978-94-009-2631-8
DOI: 10.1007/978-94-009-2631-8

**Library of Congress Cataloging in Publication Data**

Talking points in dermatology—III.

(New clinical applications. Dermatology)
Includes bibliographies and index.
1. Skin—Diseases. I. Verbov, Julian. II. Title:
Talking points in dermatology—3. III. Series.
[DNLM: 1. Skin Diseases. WR 140 T14611]
RL72.T35 1988 616.5 88–26672



Published in the United Kingdom by Kluwer Academic Publishers, PO Box 55, Lancaster, UK

Kluwer Academic Publishers BV incorporates the publishing programmes of D. Reidel, Martinus Nikhoff, Dr W. Junk and MTP Press.

# CONTENTS

# AUTHORS


*Dr A. Y. Finlay*
Senior Lecturer in Dermatology
Department of Medicine (Dermatology)
University of Wales College of Medicine
Heath Park, Cardiff
CF4 4XN

*Dr R. M. Graham*
Consultant Dermatologist
James Paget Hospital
Lowestoft Road
Great Yarmouth
NR36 6LA

*Dr R. A. C. Graham-Brown*
Consultant Dermatologist
The Leicester Royal Infirmary
Leicester
LE1 5WW

*Dr S. S. Mendelsohn*
Consultant Dermatologist
Chester Royal Infirmary
Nicholas Street
Chester
CH1 2AZ

*Dr A. G. Messenger*
Consultant Dermatologist
Royal Hallamshire Hospital
Glossop Road
Sheffield
S10 2JF

*Mr G. S. Walton*
Senior Lecturer
Department of Veterinary Clinical Science
University of Liverpool
Leahurst
Neston
S. Wirral
L64 7TE

# SERIES EDITOR'S FOREWORD

This is the ninth volume in the New Clinical Applications Dermatology Series. Some important topics that merit discussion are included in this book. Dr Messenger discusses clinicopathological aspects of the common disorder, alopecia areata. Dr Mendelsohn gives a straightforward, clear account of pregnancy eruptions. Dr Graham-Brown gives a comprehensive yet concise survey of that strange condition, lichen planus. Dr Graham treats us to a thorough appraisal of the enigmatic juvenile plantar dermatosis. Mr Walton takes an experienced comprehensive look at ectoparasites of importance to man and the concluding chapter by Dr Finlay provides a concise, helpful insight into how modern technology can aid dermatology.

JULIAN VERBOV

# ABOUT THE EDITOR

Dr Julian Verbov is Consultant Dermatologist to Liverpool Health Authority and Honorary Clinical Lecturer in Dermatology at the University of Liverpool.

He is a member of the British Association of Dermatologists, representing the British Society for Paediatric Dermatology on its Executive Committee. He is Editor of the *Proceedings of the North of England Dermatological Society*. He is a Fellow of the Zoological Society of London and a member of the Society of Authors. He is a popular national and international speaker and author of more than 200 publications. His special interests include paediatric dermatology, inherited disorders, dermatoglyphics, pruritus ani, cutaneous polyarteritis nodosa, therapeutics, drug abuse, and medical humour. He organizes the British Postgraduate Course in Paediatric Dermatology and is a member of the Editorial Board of *Clinical and Experimental Dermatology*.

# 1

# ALOPECIA AREATA

*A. G. MESSENGER*

## INTRODUCTION

The first account of alopecia areata is usually ascribed to Celsus. Writing in the first century AD, he described two patterns of hair loss under the heading 'Areae'[1]. The first, known as *alopecia* (from the Greek *alopekia* meaning 'fox-mange') '... spreads in no certain form. It is found in the hair of the head and in the beard.' The second type, known as *ophiasis*, '... begins at the hinder part of the head ... it creeps with two heads to the ears ...' However, it was not until the latter half of the nineteenth century that alopecia areata was clearly delineated from tinea capitis, and claims that alopecia areata was caused by various microorganisms continued to appear into the early years of the present century. A variety of theories as to the cause of alopecia areata have been proposed since that time. These have included endocrine dysfunction, reflex irritation and trophoneurosis. Currently, the most popular view is that alopecia areata is an autoimmune disease but, although there are grounds for believing that immunological mechanisms are involved in the disease, most of the evidence that alopecia areata is caused by autoimmunity is circumstantial. A particular problem, both in terms of understanding the aetiology and in the development of better forms of treatment, has been our poor understanding of the pathogenesis. Much research work has concentrated on various non-specific immunological abnormalities in the peripheral blood, while the target organ – the hair follicle – has been relatively neglected. This imbalance is now being corrected and this review will be devoted mainly to clinicopathological aspects of alopecia areata and to the progress that has been made in the development of model systems. Treatment will not be discussed, as this has been well reviewed recently[2].

## CLINICAL FEATURES

Alopecia areata usually presents as one or more discrete patches of hair loss. This occurs most commonly on the scalp or beard but any hair-bearing skin can be affected. The bald patches enlarge centrifugally and may coalesce. Large numbers of telogen hairs can be plucked with minimal traction from around the periphery of enlarging bald patches. The roots of these hairs may have a well-formed club or show an abnormally tapered appearance. The hair shafts often have a localized zone of weakness between 2 and 4 mm above the root. This can cause focal narrowing of the hair shaft and lead to angulation or fracture, giving rise to the characteristic 'exclamation mark' hair. The scalp itself appears normal with preservation of the follicular orifices, although there is sometimes slight erythema. Occasionally, alopecia areata presents with a diffuse hair loss. This can be difficult to differentiate from other causes of diffuse hair loss at the initial consultation, but the usual rapid course of diffuse alopecia areata, often resulting in alopecia totalis, together with other features such as exclamation mark hairs and nail changes, will usually enable the correct diagnosis to be made. Nail abnormalities occur in a small proportion of cases and are usually, though not always, associated with extensive hair loss. The exact frequency is difficult to determine and depends on what criteria are used for assessing minimal involvement. In a series collected in Sheffield by Dr R. E. Church (personal communication), 20 out of 168 cases of alopecia areata (12%) and 14 out of 30 cases of alopecia totalis (47%) showed changes in the nails. Fine stippled pitting of the nail plate is the most common finding; other changes include longitudinal ridging and roughening of the nail plate and erythema of the lunula.

The course of alopecia areata is very variable. In the majority of cases with circumscribed disease, recovery occurs within a year. The regrowing hair is fine and may be non-pigmented or hypopigmented at first. This is then replaced by progressively thicker and darker hair. In a few patients, pigmentation does not return and the regrown hair remains white. However, the course can be more prolonged. Some cases progress to total or universal alopecia and about a third of patients will still have active disease after 5 years. Even when the hair regrows, recurrences are common. Indeed, long-term follow-up studies have shown that almost all patients will experience at least one further episode of hair loss[3]. Accurate prognostication is impossible in individual patients, although the presence or absence of certain adverse risk factors may provide a guide. Generally, the chances of recovery decline as the hair loss becomes more extensive and as the duration of the disease increases. Total alopecia has a particularly poor prognosis, although some patients do recover, even from long-standing disease. The outlook is also less favourable when the onset is in childhood or in old age. The role of atopy in alopecia areata is uncertain, but atopic subjects appear to do less well than non-atopics.

## Pigmentation

There are a number of clinical features of alopecia areata that suggest that melanin pigmentation has a role in the pathogenesis.

1. There is probably an increased prevalence of vitiligo in patients with alopecia areata. There is a particularly high incidence of alopecia (70%) in the Vogt–Koyanagi–Harada syndrome, an acute inflammatory leukoderma involving skin, eyes and meninges[4].
2. Alopecia areata may occur in a perinaevoid distribution[5].
3. There may be changes in the function of retinal pigment epithelium[6].
4. Regrowing hair is frequently hypopigmented or non-pigmented.
5. In people with grey hair (which is usually a mixture of pigmented hair and white hair), alopecia areata may cause selective loss of the pigmented hair while the white hair is apparently unaffected. This is thought to be the explanation for the numerous historical accounts of rapid greying[7]. Sparing of white hair in alopecia areata is a variable phenomenon with some patients showing incomplete sparing, i.e. the white hairs appear to be more resist-

ant to the disease but are eventually lost. In a few patients, notably the elderly, white hairs are affected to the same degree as pigmented hairs.

## AETIOLOGY

### Genetic factors

The predisposition to alopecia areata is probably inherited. Published figures vary but overall suggest that 20–30% of patients with alopecia areata know of at least one other affected family member. There are also a number of case reports of alopecia areata occurring in identical and non-identical twins, sometimes with concurrent onset. In two families with a high prevalence of alopecia areata, the affected family members shared the same HLA haplotype[8,9]. The haplotype was not the same in both families (HLA-A2, B40 and HLA-Aw32, B18) and large population surveys have failed to reveal consistent linkage to any particular Class I antigens. A more recent study has suggested an association with the Class II antigen DR5[10]. The frequency of DR5 was greater in patients with severe forms of alopecia areata and an early age of onset, but the degree of association appears too low to be of major aetiological significance.

### Immunology

The idea that alopecia areata is an autoimmune disease was first proposed by Rothman in a discussion following a paper presented by Van Scott and Ekel[11]. However, most of the evidence for this hypothesis is still circumstantial. Briefly the evidence can be considered under three headings (for more detailed reviews see references 2 and 12).

### *1. Association with autoimmune diseases*

The association of alopecia areata with thyroid disease has long been recognized and was responsible for early ideas that alopecia areata is caused by endocrine dysfunction. In their series of 736 cases of alopecia areata[13], Muller and Winkelmann found 29 (8%) with thyroid disease of various types, compared with less than 2% in control subjects. An increased prevalence of thyroid disease has also been found in other series of alopecia areata, but the association is not strong and has not been confirmed by all investigators. A wide variety of other autoimmune diseases have been described in alopecia areata, though these are mainly at the anecdotal level. About 4% of patients with alopecia areata also have vitiligo[13], a prevalence probably greater than that in the general population, although whether this should be taken as evidence that alopecia areata is an autoimmune disease is somewhat debatable in view of our limited understanding of the aetiology of vitiligo.

### *2. Abnormalities of humoral immunity*

There are numerous studies of autoantibody profiles in alopecia areata. An increased frequency of organ-specific autoantibodies has been found in most, though not all, of these studies. These include antibodies against thyroid tissue, gastric parietal cells, smooth muscle, adrenal tissue and gonads. Friedmann[14] found that the prevalence of thyroid antibodies was higher in women, particularly younger women and those with alopecia totalis, whereas gastric parietal antibodies were more common in men.

### *3. Abnormalities of cellular immunity*

Although a variety of abnormalities of cellular immunity have been described in alopecia areata, a consistent pattern has not emerged. A reduction in total circulating T lymphocyte numbers has been reported in some studies, though not all, and this has been correlated with the presence of thyroid autoantibodies and with disease activity. Conflicting results have come from studies of T cell subsets where T suppressor cell numbers have been reported to be increased, normal or decreased. Lymphocyte blastogenic responses to mitogens have been normal in some studies and depressed in others. Some of these discrepancies may be due to differences in experimental techniques and patient selection. Disease 'activity' appears to be an important variable that can be difficult to assess clinically. However, it should be remembered that these types of studies are likely to reveal only very general disturbances of immune function. If cell-mediated immune responses are operating in the pathogenesis of alopecia areata, these may involve a small subset of cells with hair-follicle specificity. Their detection may require more sensitive techniques using specific antigen.

## Down's syndrome

Alopecia areata is particularly common in Down's syndrome. Du Vivier and Munro[15] found 60 cases of alopecia areata amongst 1000 patients with Down's syndrome compared with one in 1000 non-Down's mentally retarded control subjects. In the series of 214 cases of Down's syndrome reported by Carter and Jegasothy[16], there were 19 (8.9%) with alopecia areata. The reason for the increased incidence of alopecia areata in Down's syndrome is unknown, although disturbances of immune function, including autoimmunity, are common in this group.

## Atopy

The relationship between atopy and alopecia areata is uncertain, although there is general agreement that atopic subjects have a less favourable prognosis. In Ikeda's[17] series of alopecia areata cases (10% of whom were atopic), atopics showed an earlier age of onset than non-atopics. Often starting during childhood, the course tended to be prolonged and 75% progressed to total or universal alopecia. It is less clear whether alopecia areata occurs more commonly in atopics. This has been suggested by several workers, but the criteria for defining atopy have varied and control groups to which the same criteria are applied have not been studied.

### Heterogeneity

The diversity of clinical presentation and course of alopecia areata, together with the variability in disease associations and immunological abnormalities, have led to suggestions that alopecia areata is a heterogeneous disorder rather than a single disease entity[2]. The series reported by Ikeda is often quoted in this respect. She divided patients with alopecia areata into four groups:

1. A 'common' type (83%) for which the prognosis was generally good;
2. An 'atopic' type (10%) for which the prognosis was poor;
3. A 'pre-hypertensive' type (4%) who were defined as having at least one hypertensive parent and who frequently progressed to alopecia totalis;
4. An 'endocrine-autonomic' type (3%) occurring in patients over the age of 40.

With the exception of the pre-hypertensive type, this classification has been broadly accepted by other authors. Whether these findings indicate that alopecia areata represents a clinicopathological reaction pattern that may be caused by a heterogeneity of processes must await a better understanding of the nature of the hair follicle lesion. An alternative explanation is that certain aspects of the clinical course and presentation can be modified by various factors, e.g. atopy, that are not directly related to specific causal factors.

## PATHOGENESIS

### The normal hair follicle

From a functional point of view, the hair follicle can be divided into an upper 'permanent' region above the level of the arrector insertion and a lower 'transient' region. Anatomically, the permanent region, comprising the infundibulum, the sebaceous apparatus and the isthmus, is a relatively static structure. The lower part of the hair follicle, however, undergoes major structural changes during the course of the hair cycle. Alopecia areata appears to be a disorder of the transient region and an appreciation of certain salient aspects of the normal anatomy and physiology is important in understanding the pathological changes that occur in various stages of the disease.

The structure of an anagen hair bulb is represented in Figure 1.1. Cells at the base of the bulb comprise the epithelial matrix, the proliferative population of cells from which the inner root sheath and the hair shaft are derived. As cells move away from the matrix they differentiate in a highly ordered fashion to form the Henley layer, Huxley layer and cuticle of the inner root sheath and the cuticle, cortex and medulla of the hair shaft. There are no specific markers that will indicate the ultimate destiny of an individual matrix cell. However, by following the differentiated compartments back to the matrix, it appears that the inner root sheath is derived from cells in the lower bulb, whereas the hair cortex arises from more distal cells, henceforth referred to as the 'pre-cortical matrix', situated around the central and (in non-medullated follicles) the upper part of the dermal papilla. At

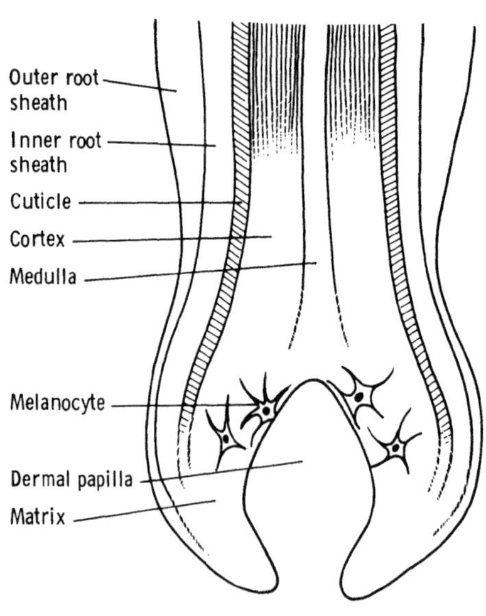


FIGURE 1.1 Diagram of the normal anagen hair bulb

the level of the matrix, the outer root sheath consists of a single layer of cells that can be followed almost to the lower tip of the bulb. Distal to the hair bulb, the outer root sheath becomes multi-layered. It is not yet clear whether matrix activity contributes to the outer root sheath (or vice versa).

Hair growth is not continuous. Each follicle undergoes repetitive sequences of growth (anagen) and rest (telogen) known as the hair cycle. Between anagen and telogen there is a brief involutional phase known as catagen. As will be seen later, the development of the anagen follicle is particularly relevant to the pathogenesis of alopecia areata. The sub-division of anagen development into six stages by Chase and his colleagues[18] is generally accepted and is illustrated in Figure 1.2. The duration of anagen is variable depending on body site. On the scalp, anagen lasts between 2 and 5 years. Hair growth then declines and finally ceases as the follicle enters the involutional phase of catagen before returning to telogen.

We have only a limited understanding of the regulatory mechanisms responsible for controlling the hair cycle. In some mammals hair cycles are coordinated, but in man individual hair follicles cycle independently of their neighbours. Although systemic factors, such as hormones, may influence the duration of the various phases of the cycle, the major regulatory factors must be intrinsic to each follicle. Embryologically, the hair follicle is derived from both ectodermal and mesenchymal tissue. The mesenchymal component, which will ultimately form the dermal papilla and the fibrous sheath around the follicle, appears as a condensation of cells intimately associated with a group of overlying epidermal cells from which the hair follicle epithelium will arise. The cellular population of the papilla is established early in the course of follicular morphogenesis and the papilla thereafter persists as a discrete structure associated with the base of the follicle throughout successive adult hair cycles. It has long been known that differentiation of hair follicles from foetal epidermis is dependent on inductive stimuli derived from the mesenchyme. Anagen development in the adult follicle closely resembles embryonic development and there is compelling evidence that the dermal papilla is also responsible for inducing hair matrix differentiation in adult life[19,20]. During the course of the hair cycle, major changes can be observed within the papilla in terms of cellular morphology and composition

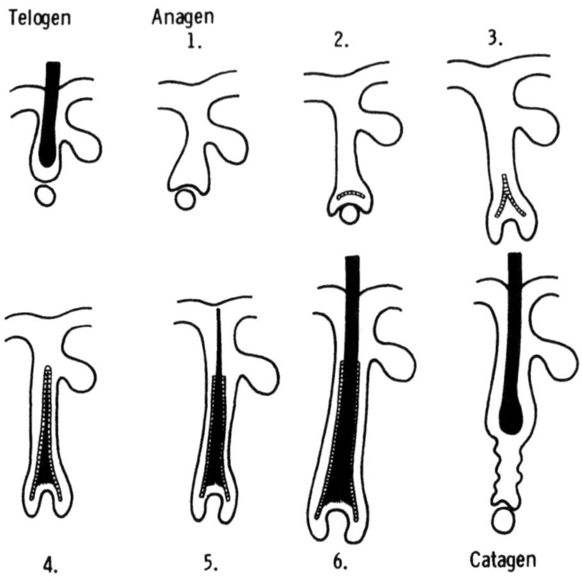


FIGURE 1.2 The hair cycle. The 6 stages of anagen development are illustrated. *Anagen 1:* There is onset of mitotic activity in the secondary germ, which grows down to invest the dermal papilla. *Anagen 2:* The inner root sheath appears as a plate of keratinized cells (hatched) overlying the developing epithelial matrix. *Anagen 3:* The inner root sheath has extended to form a conical structure beneath which the cortex has started to differentiate but is not yet keratinizing. *Anagen 4:* The cortex is now keratinized. *Anagen 5:* The hair cortex penetrates the inner root sheath at the level of the sebaceous duct. *Anagen 6:* The fully developed anagen follicle. The telogen hair is not usually lost until Anagen 5 or 6 but, for clarity, this is omitted from the diagram

of the extracellular matrix, but the nature of the inductive signals to the hair bulb epithelium is not yet known.

Two other cell types, melanocytes and Langerhans cells, are found within hair bulb epithelium. During anagen, melanocytes reside amongst cells of the pre-cortical matrix around the upper half of the dermal papilla. Pigment is donated almost exclusively to cells undergoing early cortical differentiation, although occasionally pigment is also seen in the cuticle and the medulla. Small numbers of inactive melanocytes can be found in the secondary germ region of telogen follicles. These cells accompany the hair bulb as it starts to differentiate in early anagen but do not begin to synthesize tyrosinase and melanin until Anagen 3. There is a concomitant increase in melanocyte numbers at this stage. Pigment transfer to cortical keratinocytes begins in Anagen 4 and continues until catagen approaches. A decline in pigment transfer is an early indicator of catagen occurring before other morphological changes and this ceases altogether during catagen itself. Very little is known about the regulation of melanocyte activity in the hair follicle. However, the close anatomical and functional relationship between hair bulb melanocytes and cortical keratinocytes suggests that activation of pigmentary activity may be dependent on stimuli emanating from the principal receptor cell, i.e. the cortical keratinocyte. Langerhans cells are also found in the hair bulb although only in very low numbers. Their function in this site is unknown.

## Pathodynamics

Alopecia areata is a four-dimensional disease, not only in the sense that any inflammatory disorder has a time course, but also because it alters the dynamics of the hair cycle. This is important, firstly because it causes difficulties in the interpretation of histological material and, secondly, because an understanding of the pathodynamic changes may provide clues to the nature of the hair follicle pathology.

The most detailed study of the early changes in alopecia areata was that carried out by Eckert and her colleagues[21]. They determined anagen–telogen ratios in hairs plucked from demarcated concentric zones around the periphery of enlarging bald patches. Loss of hair was preceded by a large increase in the proportion of telogen hairs. There was also an increase in the number of anagen hairs showing dystrophic features. They concluded that the initial event was a precipitation of anagen follicles into telogen. Less severely affected follicles may remain in anagen for a time but these would produce a dystrophic hair and eventually would also undergo telogen conversion. These findings have been supported by histological studies[22,23]. Biopsies taken from the edges of expanding bald patches show that the majority of follicles are in various stages of catagen and early telogen (Figure 1.3). It is not clear whether follicles attain telogen via normal catagen. Exclamation mark hairs may have a well-formed club root identical to that of a normal telogen hair. However, the root is frequently narrowed and dystrophic and club hairs from around alopecic lesions fall out more readily than normally, suggesting that there is defective anchoring within the follicle. Headington and co-workers[23] maintain that catagen is abnormal in alopecia areata and used the term 'nanogen' to describe this, although they have yet to publish their findings in full.

Although there is some uncertainty as to how it is achieved, there

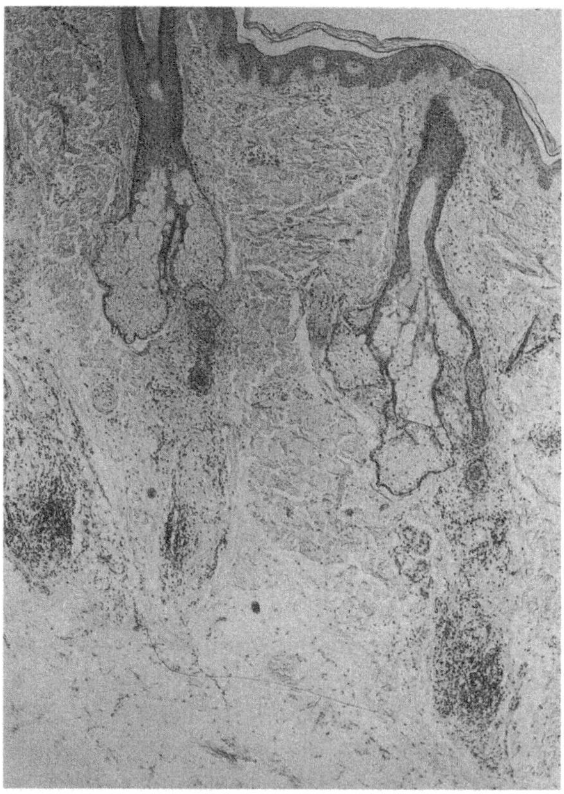

FIGURE 1.3 Alopecia areata. The biopsy is from the edge of an expanding lesion and shows two follicles in late catagen. There is a lymphocytic infiltrate deep in the dermis at the site occupied by the hair bulbs when in anagen ( × 40)

is general agreement that follicles undergo telogen conversion in the initial stages of alopecia areata. However, there are conflicting views as to what happens next. Swanson and his colleagues[24] have stated that alopecia areata causes arrest of follicles in telogen This is contrary to the findings published previously by Van Scott[25]. He studied biopsies taken from bald patches and found an average of 58% of follicles in anagen, suggesting re-entry into anagen after the initial telogen conversion. In early lesions, there was a reduction in the size of the transient region with preservation of the upper part of the follicle and the sebaceous gland. In long-standing disease, the entire follicle became smaller. The matrix region of these miniaturized anagen fol-

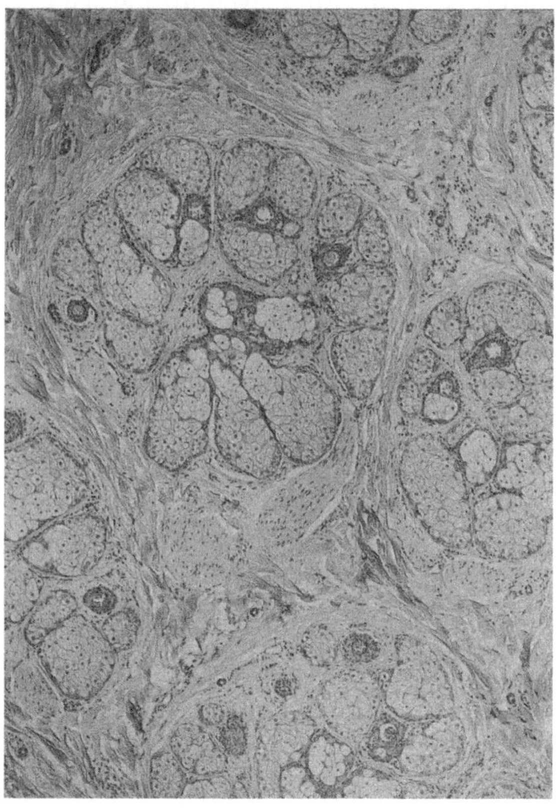

FIGURE 1.4 Alopecia totalis of one year's duration. Horizontal section at the level of sebaceous glands showing normal follicle numbers ( × 40)

licles was mitotically active and produced a normal inner root sheath. However, the cortex was incompletely keratinized. Van Scott interpreted these changes as indicating arrest of development in Anagen 4. We[22] have broadly confirmed the findings of Van Scott. Biopsies taken from established bald patches and from alopecia totalis were examined using serial horizontal sections. Total follicle numbers were within normal limits in 7 of the 8 patients studied (Figure 1.4) and anagen follicles, in proportions varying between 16% and 62%, were always demonstrable. However, none showed development beyond Anagen 3 (Figure 1.5). As a follicle could not remain indefinitely in Anagen 3 (continued matrix activity would inevitably lead to progressive lengthening of the cortex and penetration of the inner root sheath), it must then return prematurely to telogen for the same sequence to be repeated. It is probable that these truncated cycles continue until such time as the disease activity subsides (Figure 1.6).

## Immunopathology

A peribulbar lymphocytic infiltrate is a constant feature of alopecia areata. Lymphocytes also infiltrate the dermal papilla and the hair bulb and outer root-sheath epithelium. This is seen mainly in association with anagen follicles and is scanty around telogen bulbs. The density of the infiltrate is very variable. Generally, it tends to be more prominent in early lesions, whereas in long-standing alopecia totalis the infiltrate can be quite sparse. An inflammatory infiltrate may also

FIGURE 1.5 Alopecia areata. Serial horizontal sections from an established bald patch through a single anagen follicle. (**a**) Matrix level. The dermal papilla is in the centre of the follicle and there is a peribulbar lymphocytic infiltrate. (**b**) Section taken just above the upper pole of the dermal papilla. There is a single cell peripheral layer of outer root sheath within which is the keratinizing inner root sheath. The cortex is in the centre of the follicle but is not keratinized. (**c**) Distal to level (**b**) the outer root sheath is multilayered. The keratinized inner root sheath is continuous over the centre of the follicle.

In three dimensions the inner root sheath would be conical in shape. The cortex is starting to differentiate but is not keratinized. This stage of development is equivalent to Anagen 3. ORS, outer root sheath; IRS, inner root sheath; C, Cortex; DP, dermal papilla ( × 250)

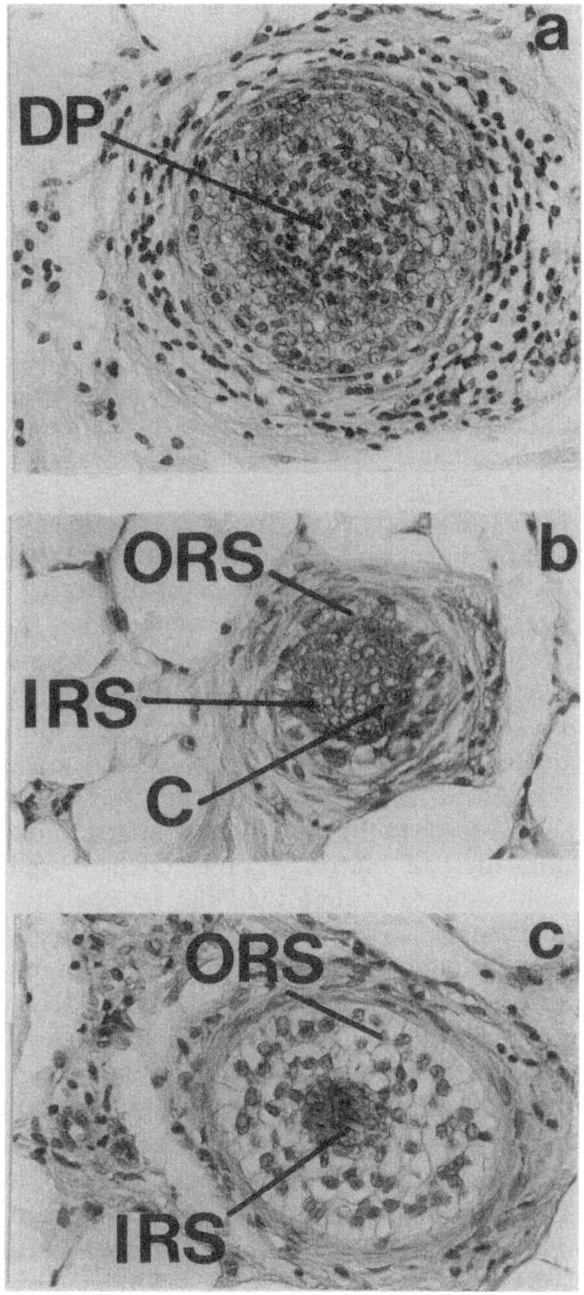
a
DP
b
ORS
IRS
C
c
ORS
IRS

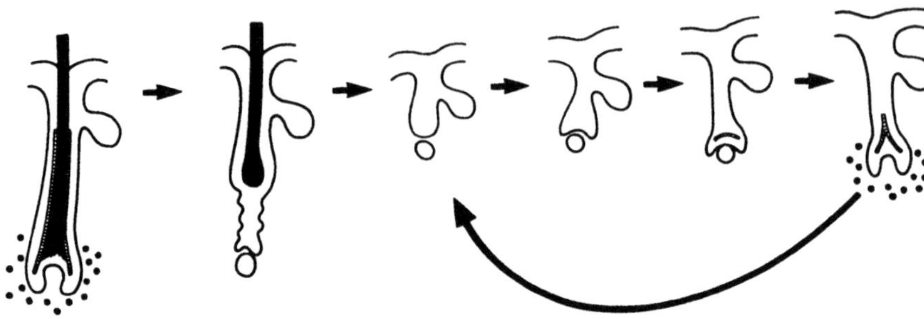

FIGURE 1.6 Proposed pathodynamic changes in alopecia areata. The initial event is telogen conversion. There is re-entry into anagen, but development is halted in Anagen 3 and the follicle returns to telogen. Repeated cycling to Anagen 3 continues until the disease activity subsides

be seen around the upper part of the follicle together with spongiosis of infundibular epithelium. The relevance of this to the pathogenesis of alopecia areata is obscure, as similar changes are found in male-pattern alopecia and sometimes in normal scalp. Immunohistochemical studies using monoclonal antibodies have shown that the peribulbar and intrabulbar infiltrate mostly comprises HLA-DR positive (activated) T lymphocytes with a helper:suppressor ratio of around 3:1[26,27]. Dendritic cells bearing the OKT6 Langerhans cell marker may also be seen in the perifollicular infiltrate and in increased numbers within the hair bulb[28]. Whether OKT6+ cells are indeed Langerhans cells needs to be confirmed ultrastructurally. Monoclonal antibody studies have also revealed that there is altered expression of major histocompatibility complex (MHC) antigens by hair-follicle epithelium. In normal skin, Class I MHC antigens (HLA-A, B, C) are expressed on keratinocyte cell membranes in the epidermis and in the permanent region of the hair follicle. Below the level of the arrector insertion, outer root sheath cells do not express Class I antigens. Some investigators have also found absence of Class I expression in matrix epithelium, although others have demonstrated weak expression by these cells[29,30]. This discrepancy could be due to differences in antibody affinities or in the sensitivity of the immunohistochemical techniques. The expression of the Class II antigen, HLA-DR, is normally confined to dendritic cells, presumably Langerhans cells. These are very sparse in the lower follicle, being found in only low numbers in the matrix region. However, in lesional areas of alopecia areata, 50–70% of anagen follicles display expression of HLA-DR by epithelial cells[31]. Expression of HLA-DR occurs mainly on matrix cells around the upper pole of the dermal papilla, i.e. the precortical matrix, and in the presumptive cortex (Figure 1.7). Aberrant expression of HLA-DR, by cells that are normally HLA-DR negative, occurs in a wide variety of disorders characterized by lymphocytic infiltrates containing activated T-cells[32]. Activated T cells release cytokines, such as $\gamma$-interferon which can induce HLA-DR expression in various cell types *in vitro*, but whether this phenomenon is of any pathobiological significance is uncertain. Bottazzo and his colleagues[33] have suggested that increased HLA-DR expression is a primary event in autoimmune disease. They proposed that, in genetically predisposed individuals, increased HLA-DR expression would occur in response to various non-specific stimuli, such as viral infections, and facilitate the presentation of autoantigens to helper T-cells. This seems unlikely in alopecia areata, because HLA-DR expression appears to be a late event and is not seen in non-lesional or perilesional follicles[27]. Alternative possibilities include a role in perpetuating or downgrading an immune reaction. Recently, it has also been shown that there is also increased expression of Class I antigens in the matrix region of anagen follicles from alopecia areata[29]. The distribution of Class I expression was similar to that of Class II expression. Class I antigens are necessary for the recognition of antigen by primed cytotoxic T-cells and increased expression could therefore enhance a putative cell-mediated immune assault on the hair follicle.

Whatever the precise significance of these observations in terms of the pathogenesis of alopecia areata, the altered hair follicle MHC expression strongly suggests that an immune mechanism is involved in the generation of the follicular lesion although, at present, we can only speculate as to its nature. The absence of B-cells within the follicular infiltrate[27] argues against an antibody-mediated lesion. Direct and indirect immunofluorescence studies have failed to reveal evidence of hair follicle antibodies, although not all autoantibodies can be demonstrated by these techniques (e.g. TSH receptor antibodies in Graves' disease). Nunzi and colleagues[34] claimed to have eluted immunoglobulin from lymphocytes of patients with alopecia areata that bound to the perifollicular capillaries, but this finding has yet to

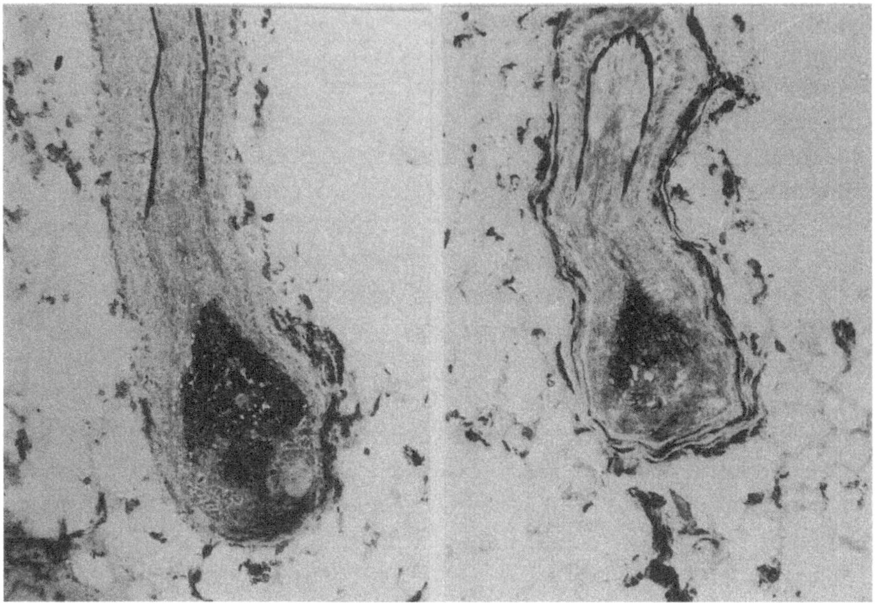

FIGURE 1.7 Anagen follicles from alopecia areata stained for HLA-DR (immunoperoxidase). There is intense staining in the precortical matrix and presumptive cortex. Staining of inner root sheath is with Toluidine Blue ( × 100)

be confirmed by others. On present evidence, a cell-mediated cytotoxic assault appears the most likely explanation, though the absence of suitable sources of putative antigen has made specific cellular hypersensitivity difficult to test and the possibility that the cellular infiltrate is a secondary phenomenon cannot be excluded.

## Hair follicle pathology

The altered hair cycle dynamics and the distribution of the immunopathological changes indicate that alopecia areata is a disorder of the transient region of the hair follicle. Can the disease target be identified more precisely? Information on this topic is limited, but two schools of thought have evolved.

### *1. Hair follicle mesenchyme as the disease target*

In view of the important role played by the dermal papilla in inducing hair-matrix differentiation, the idea that alopecia areata is primarily a disorder of the mesenchymal component of the follicle merits consideration. The main evidence for this is as follows.

(i) In a detailed morphometric study, Van Scott and Ekel[11] showed that there is a constant relationship between the volume of the dermal papilla and the volume of the epithelial matrix in normal anagen follicles. The ratio between the number of cells in the papilla and the number of mitoses in the matrix is also constant and this is maintained in the miniaturized follicles of androgenetic alopecia. However, in alopecia areata, although there is a reduction in the overall size of the papilla, the ratios between papilla volume and matrix volume and between the numbers of papilla cells and matrix mitoses are increased. They suggested that the epithelial changes were secondary to dysfunction of the dermal papilla.

(ii) Pierard and de la Brassinne[35] studied proliferative activity in the normal rat follicle during the hair cycle and in normal human follicles that had been induced to enter early anagen by plucking. DNA synthesis in the dermal papilla, as determined by [$^3$H]thymidine labelling and autoradiography, occurred predominantly during the Anagen 4 stage of development. Although the nature of their histological material prevented precise identification of the site of DNA synthesis, they felt this was mostly in endothelial cells and mast cells rather than papilla fibroblasts. They used a similar method to study biopsies from alopecia areata[36]. Little or no labelling was seen in the dermal papilla of follicles arrested in Anagen 4. Furthermore, during early regrowth, recovery of DNA synthesis in the dermal papilla appeared to precede that in the epithelial matrix. From these two studies, the authors surmised that a critical event occurs in hair follicle connective tissue during Anagen 4 and that this is impaired in alopecia areata, resulting in arrest of development at this stage. This was the first attempt to relate the hair follicle pathology in alopecia areata to the pathodynamic changes. It is possible that the changes observed were secondary to the disturbance of the hair cycle. However, further work in this area is warranted and should be facilitated by the recent development of methods for culturing cells from human dermal papillae.

*2. Epithelial matrix as the disease target*

We can infer from the exclamation mark hair that alopecia areata damages hair follicle epithelium. The focal weakness that results in fracture of the hair occurs because of injury to cells in the hair-bulb matrix and the presumptive cortex. This was first noted by Thies[37], who described vacuolar degeneration of matrix cells overlying the upper pole of the dermal papilla (Figure 1.8). These findings have been confirmed in a more recent electron microscopic study in which cell injury was observed in the precortical matrix and presumptive cortex of anagen follicles from lesional areas[38]. The features of cell injury were non-specific, although lymphocytes were seen infiltrating the hair bulb in keeping with an immunocytotoxic mechanism. Matrix injury could be secondary to pathology occurring in the connective

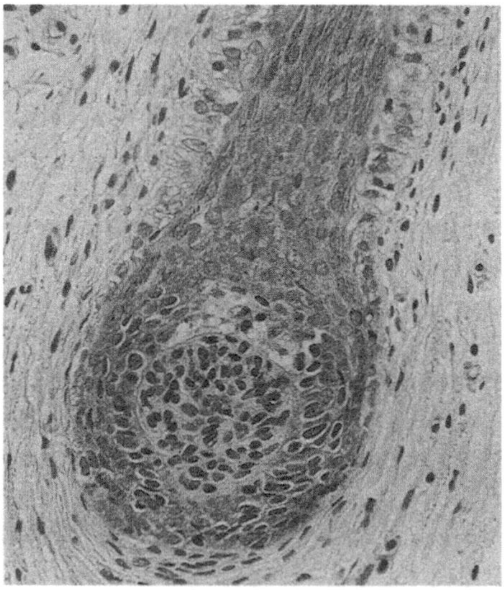

FIGURE 1.8 Early anagen follicle from alopecia totalis. There is vacuolation in the precortical matrix overlying the upper pole of the dermal papilla ( × 100)

tissue compartment. However, the possibility that cells undergoing early cortical differentiation form the primary target can be supported by the following observations:

1. Cell injury is not seen in other differentiating compartments such as the inner root sheath. Unless there is a specific interaction between papilla and pre-cortical matrix it seems unlikely that cell injury secondary to papilla dysfunction would be so selective.
2. These cells frequently display aberrant expression of MHC antigens.
3. The pathodynamic changes can be explained on this basis. The initial telogen conversion provides a means whereby the follicle can protect itself from further injury. Whilst it is in telogen the follicle is 'safe', as no differentiative activity is occurring. Re-entry into anagen can take place unhindered, but as soon as cortex starts to develop (in Anagen 3) the attack is resumed. The ability of the follicle to return to telogen from this stage may explain why follicles are not destroyed in alopecia areata.

The various pigmentary features have recently given rise to renewed interest in a third possibility, i.e. that alopecia areata is primarily a disorder affecting hair-bulb melanocytes. Melanocytes cannot be found in senile white hair bulbs and this idea would seem to provide an explanation for the sparing of white hair. However, unless we introduce the concept of heterogeneity, this is difficult to sustain as sparing of white hair is not a consistent finding. We studied the effect of alopecia areata on hair pigmentation by electron microscopy of regrowing white hair bulbs[38]. Most of these follicles contained small numbers of melanocytes. Melanosomes were scanty and poorly melanized and there was no evidence of pigment transfer to cortical keratinocytes. However, melanocyte ultrastructure was well-preserved even where there was severe injury to adjacent keratinocytes. We surmised that the pigmentary changes were secondary to keratinocyte injury, but a better appreciation of how melanocyte activity is regulated in the hair follicle will be necessary before they can be fully understood. Although the reason for the sparing of white hairs in alopecia areata remains elusive, an interesting analogy can be drawn with vitiligo. Recently, it has been shown that, in previously sensitized individuals, vitiliginous skin is less responsive than normally pigmented skin to epicutaneous challenge with contact allergens[39,40]. This intriguing phenomenon suggests that there is a link between susceptibility to cell-mediated immune reactions in keratinocyte populations and pigmentation.

## MODELS FOR ALOPECIA AREATA

The absence of suitable model systems has considerably restricted the scope of research into the biology and pathology of human hair growth. Tissue sections can provide information about morphological change, but what this means in terms of function may be open to more than one interpretation. However, advances are now being made in the development of various models for studying both normal hair growth and alopecia areata.

### Cell culture

Progress has been made in culturing cells derived from the epithelial and dermal compartments of the hair follicle[41]. Isolated dermal papillae can be cultured from a variety of mammalian species, including man, and the cells can be maintained for prolonged periods in the laboratory. These cells display a number of characteristic features in terms of their morphology, behaviour and synthetic activity, which resemble those of the parent tissue. Cells cultured from the rat-whisker dermal papilla also retain the ability to induce hair growth when reimplanted into the intact animal[42]. This inductive property has not yet been demonstrated in human dermal papilla cells, although so far this has only been tested *in vitro*. Epithelial cells can be cultured from the outer root sheath of plucked human follicles, though they show an epidermoid growth pattern *in vitro* and do not form matrix-like structures. Culture techniques are still at an early stage of development and, at present, we cannot obtain cells that display features of epithelial matrix differentiation. Further work is also required to establish to what extent cultured cells retain their *in vivo* properties before these techniques can be reliably applied to the study of alopecia areata.

## The nude mouse

The nude mouse is unable to mount a graft rejection response because it lacks a functioning thymus. This trait has been of great value in studying cellular immunity and has recently been applied to alopecia areata. Gilhar and Krueger transplanted 2 mm punch biopsies, complete with hair follicles, from the scalp of patients with alopecia universalis and alopecia areata onto nude mice[43]. After 48 days, hair growth was present in many surviving grafts. Curiously, hair growth was better in grafts taken from patients with alopecia universalis than those from alopecia areata. These important findings suggest that circulating factors, present in the human subject but not in the nude mouse, were responsible for causing the follicular lesion. The same authors also showed that systemic administration of cyclosporin, a drug that stimulates normal hair growth in man, would enhance regrowth in the transplants. Cyclosporin has been used topically to treat alopecia areata. The results are not very inspiring, but it is doubtful whether there is significant absorption by this route. Most physicians would be reluctant to administer cyclosporin systemically for alopecia areata because of its nephrotoxicity, but the results in the nude mouse model should stimulate a search for analogues that can be absorbed topically.

## The DEBR rat

The DEBR rat appeared as a spontaneous mutation in the animal house of Dundee University[44]. DEBR rats grow an apparently normal first coat of hair after birth and then become progressively hairless. Histologically, follicles are present and show a perifollicular and intrafollicular lymphocytic infiltrate. There is also vacuolar degeneration in the cortex of anagen follicles. Regrowth of hair can be stimulated by PUVA and by topical application of minoxidil. PUVA-induced regrowth was restricted to the exposed areas but in minoxidil-treated rats hair growth occurred over the whole body and was not limited to the sites of application. These features resemble human alopecia areata quite closely, although the response to treatment is perhaps more impressive than that seen in clinical practice. Another interesting feature of this animal is that alopecic skin will regrow hair when transplanted onto athymic nude mice, again implicating a circulating factor in the pathogenesis.

## CONCLUSIONS

The treatment of alopecia areata is unsatisfactory. Although there are treatments that will stimulate hair growth, none alters the natural history and the results in terms of cosmesis are often poor. If we are to develop better treatments we need to know more about the biology of normal hair growth and how this is altered by the disease. It seems likely that immunological mechanisms are involved in the pathogenesis of alopecia areata, but there is no conclusive evidence that an autoimmune process is operating and we should be prepared to consider other possibilities. For example, could immunological factors, e.g. cytokines, be involved in regulating normal hair growth and alopecia areata represent a derangement of this system? Understanding what happens in the hair follicle itself will be of crucial importance and it is hoped that the application of new techniques, such as the use of cell culture and animal models, will provide the means to this end. At the same time it should be possible to use these models in the development and testing of new forms of treatment.

### Acknowledgements

Figures 1.1, 1.2, 1.3, 1.4, 1.5 and 1.8 are reprinted with the permission of the *British Journal of Dermatology*. Figure 1.7 is reprinted with the permission of the *Journal of Investigative Dermatology*.

## REFERENCES

1. Celsus, A. C. (1838). In *Of Medicine*, Book VI, pp. 292–293 (translated by James Grieve), (London: H. Renshaw)
2. Mitchell, A. J. and Balle, M. R. (1987). Alopecia areata. *Dermatol. Clin.*, **5**, 553–564
3. Walker, S. A. and Rothman, S. (1950). Alopecia areata. A statistical study and

consideration of endocrine influences. *J. Invest. Dermatol.*, **14,** 403–413
4. Rosen, E. (1945). Uveitis with poliosis, vitiligo, alopecia and dysacousia (Vogt-Koyanagi-Harada syndrome). *Arch. Ophthalmol.*, **33,** 281–292
5. Yesudian, P. and Thambiah, A. S. (1976). Perinevoid alopecia. An unusual variety of alopecia areata. *Arch. Dermatol.*, **112,** 1432–1434
6. Tosti, A., Colombati, S., De Padova, M. P., Guidi, S. G., Tosti, G. and Maccolini, E. (1986). Retinal pigment epithelium function in alopecia areata. *J. Invest. Dermatol.*, **86,** 553–555
7. Jelinek, J. E. (1972). Sudden whitening of the hair. *Bull. NY Acad. Med.*, **48,** 1003–1013
8. Hordinsky, M. K., Hallgren, H., Nelson, D. *et al.* (1984). Familial alopecia areata: HLA antigens and autoantibody in an American family. *Arch. Dermatol.*, **120,** 464–468
9. Valsecchi, R., Vicari, O., Frigeni, A., Foiadelli, L., Naldi, L. and Cainelli, T. (1985). Familial alopecia areata—genetic susceptibility or coincidence? *Acta Dermatol; Venereol.*, (*Stockh.*) **65,** 175–177
10. Orecchia, G., Cuccia Belvedere, M., Martinetti, M., Capelli, E. and Rabbiosi, G. (1987). Human leukocyte antigen region involvement in the genetic predisposition to alopecia areata. *Dermatologica*, **175,** 10–14
11. Van Scott, E. J. and Ekel, T. (1958). Geometric relationships between the matrix of the hair bulb and its dermal papilla in normal and alopecic scalp. *J. Invest. Dermatol.*, **31,** 281–287
12. Editorial (1984). Alopecia areata—an autoimmune disease? *Lancet*, **1,** 1335–1336
13. Muller, S. A. and Winkelmann, R. K. (1963). Alopecia areata. *Arch. Dermatol.*, **88,** 290–297
14. Friedmann, P. S. (1981). Alopecia areata and autoimmunity. *Br. J. Dermatol.*, **105,** 153–157
15. Du Vivier, A. and Munro, D. D. (1975). Alopecia areata, autoimmunity and Down syndrome. *Br. Med. J.*, **1,** 191–192
16. Carter, D. M. and Jegasothy, B. V. (1976). Alopecia areata and Down's syndrome. *Arch. Dermatol.*, **112,** 1397–1399
17. Ikeda, T. (1965). A new classification of alopecia areata. *Dermatologica*, **131,** 421–445
18. Chase, H. B., Rauch, H. and Smith, V. W. (1951). Critical stages of hair development and pigmentation in the mouse. *Physiol. Zool.*, **24,** 1–8
19. Oliver, R. F. (1967). The experimental induction of whisker growth in the hooded rat by implantation of dermal papillae. *J. Embryol. Exp. Morphol.*, **18,** 43–51
20. Oliver, R. F. (1970). The induction of hair follicle formation in the adult hooded rat by vibrissa dermal papillae. *J. Embryol. Exp. Morphol.*, **23,** 219–236
21. Eckert, J., Church, R. E. and Ebling, F. J. (1968). The pathogenesis of alopecia areata. *Br. J. Dermatol.*, **80,** 203–210
22. Messenger, A. G., Slater, D. N. and Bleehen, S. S. (1986). Alopecia areata: alterations in the hair growth cycle and correlation with the follicular pathology. *Br. J. Dermatol.*, **114,** 337–347
23. Headington, J. T., Mitchell, A. and Swanson, N. (1981). New histopathologic findings in alopecia areata studied in transverse section. *J. Invest. Dermatol.*, **76,** 325
24. Swanson, N. A., Mitchell, A. J., Leahy, M. S., Headington, J. T. and Diaz, L. A. (1981). Topical treatment of alopecia areata. Contact allergen vs primary irritant therapy. *Arch. Dermatol.*, **117,** 384–387

25. Van Scott, E. J. (1958). Morphologic changes in pilosebaceous units and anagen hairs in alopecia areata. *J. Invest. Dermatol.*, **31,** 35–43
26. Perret, C., Wiesner-Menzel, L. and Happle, R. (1984). Immunohistochemical analysis of T-cell subsets in the peribulbar and intrabulbar infiltrates of alopecia areata. *Acta Dermatol. Venereol.* (*Stockh.*) **64,** 26–30
27. Peeroboom-Wynia, J. D. R., Van Joost, T., Stolz, E. and Prins, M. E. F. (1986). Markers of immunologic injury in progressive alopecia areata. *J. Cutan. Pathol.*, **13,** 363–369
28. Wiesner-Menzel, L. and Happle, R. (1984). Intrabulbar and peribulbar accumulation of dendritic OKT6-positive cells in alopecia areata. *Arch. Dermatol. Res.*, **276,** 333–334
29. Brocker, E., Echternacht-Happle, K., Hamm, H. and Happle, R. (1987). Abnormal expression of Class I and Class II major histocompatibility antigens in alopecia areata: modulation by topical immunotherapy. *J. Invest. Dermatol.*, **88,** 564–568
30. Messenger, A. G., Romani, N. and Fritsch, P. (1983). Beta-2 microglobulin and Langerhans cells in the human anagen hair follicle. *Br. J. Dermatol.*, **109,** 713–714
31. Messenger, A. G. and Bleehen, S. S. (1985). Expression of HLA-DR by anagen hair follicles in alopecia areata. *J. Invest. Dermatol.*, **85,** 569–572
32. Aubock, J., Romani, N., Grubauer, G. and Fritsch, P. (1986). HLA-DR expression on keratinocytes is a common feature of diseased skin. *Br. J. Dermatol.*, **114,** 465–472
33. Bottazzo, G. F., Pujol-Borrell, R., Hanafusa, T. and Feldmann, M. (1983). Role of aberrant HLA-DR expression and antigen presentation in induction of endocrine autoimmunity. *Lancet*, **ii,** 1115–1119
34. Nunzi, E., Hamerlinck, F. and Cormane, R. H. (1980). Immunopathological studies on alopecia areata. *Arch. Dermatol., Res.* **269,** 1–11
35. Pierard, G. E. and De La Brassinne, M. (1975). Modulation of dermal cell activity during hair growth in the rat. *J. Cutan. Pathol.*, **2,** 35–41
36. Pierard, G. E. and De La Brassinne, M. (1975). Cellular activity in the dermis surrounding the hair bulb in alopecia areata. *J. Cutan. Pathol.*, **2,** 240–245
37. Thies, M. (1966). Vergleichende histologische Untersuchungen bei Alopecia areata und narbig-atrophisierenden Alopecien. *Archiv fur klinische und experimentelle Dermatologie*, **227,** 541–549
38. Messenger, A. G. and Bleehen, S. S. (1984). Alopecia areata: light and electron microscopic pathology of the regrowing white hair. *Br. J. Dermatol.*, **110,** 155–162
39. Uehara, M., Miyauchi, H. and Tanaka, S. (1984). Diminished contact sensitivity response in vitiliginous skin. *Arch. Dermatol.*, **120,** 195–198
40. Nordlund, J., Forget, B., Kirkwood, J. and Lerner, A. B. (1985). Dermatitis produced by applications of monobenzone in patients with active vitiligo. *Arch. Dermatol.*, **121,** 1141–1144
41. Messenger, A. G. (1985). Hair follicle tissue culture. *Br. J. Dermatol.*, **113,** 639–640
42. Jahoda, C. A. B., Horne, K. A. and Oliver, R. F. (1984). Induction of hair growth by implantation of cultured dermal papilla cells. *Nature*, **311,** 560–562
43. Gilhar, A. and Krueger, G. G. (1987). Hair growth in scalp grafts from patients

with alopecia areata and alopecia universalis grafted onto nude mice. *Arch. Dermatol.*, **123**, 44–50
44. Horne, K. A., Jahoda, C. A. B., Johnson, B. E., Michie, H. J. and Oliver, R. F. (1987). An animal model for alopecia. *J. Invest. Dermatol.*, **89**, 316

# 2

# PREGNANCY ERUPTIONS

*S. S. MENDELSOHN*

Pregnancy exerts profound changes in many of the body's systems and so it is hardly surprising that its effects on the skin are so wide ranging. It is simplest to divide these changes into three main groups.

- Physiological skin changes
- The effect of pregnancy of skin disorders
- Specific dermatoses of pregnancy

## PHYSIOLOGICAL SKIN CHANGES

Physiological skin changes in pregnancy include the following.

- Hyperpigmentation
- Vascular changes
- Changes in the oral mucosa
- Changes in the hair
- Striae distensae
- Pruritus gravidarum

### Hyperpigmentation

Hyperpigmentation in pregnancy is extremely common, affecting up to 90% of women and tending to occur early in pregnancy in the first trimester[1]. Dark-haired individuals are particularly affected. Although disputed, it is suggested that the pigmentation is due to the hormones oestrogen and progesterone, which are known to be strong melanogenic stimulants. The role of MSH in producing pregnancy hyperpigmentation is unclear.

In pregnancy, normally hyperpigmented regions may become accentuated in addition to the development of the linea nigra. These changes fade after delivery but seldom return to normal levels of pigmentation.

One of the best known changes is melasma (syn. chloasma), sometimes called the mask of pregnancy, with well-demarcated symmetrical macular pigmentation of the face. This can affect up to 75% of women and tends to present in the second half of pregnancy. The commonest of the three patterns is known as the centrofacial pattern, with pigmentation involving the cheeks, forehead, upper lip, nose and chin[2]. The malar and mandibular patterns are less common. Sunlight can exacerbate the development of melasma. Although melasma usually disappears within a year of delivery, it can often persist. Treatment with a depigmenting agent such as 5% hydroquinone in aqueous cream can be tried, but often with disappointing results, particularly if the melanin deposition is predominantly dermal.

Recently, a new physiological change of pregnancy has been described. This is the development during pregnancy of group B pigmentary demarcation lines. These lines can occur as a natural phenomenon in dark-skinned individuals. Group B lines start at the perineum and run towards the popliteal fossae and can extend as far as the ankles. Vázquez *et al.*[3] describe four women who developed these lines for the first time during pregnancy. In all four cases the lines faded postpartum.

## Vascular changes

The two commonest vascular changes to occur in pregnancy are the development of spider naevi and palmar erythema. These can affect up to two thirds of pregnant women. Both these changes are probably due to the effect of oestrogens and the hyperkinetic circulation of pregnancy may also contribute.

Spider naevi appear during the second to fifth months of pregnancy, usually in the areas drained by the superior vena cava. Palmar ery-

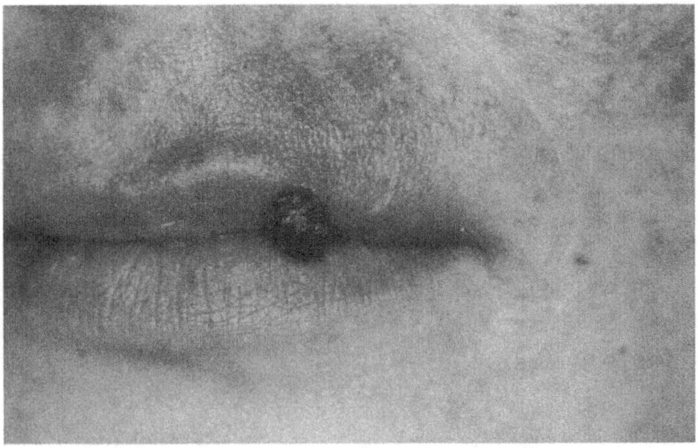

FIGURE 2.1 Haemangioma occurring in pregnancy that required curettage and cautery

thema appears a little earlier. Both these phenomena regress after delivery and no treatment is required.

Cutaneous haemangiomata can develop in up to 5% of women and usually appear towards the end of the first trimester. Although they tend to resolve after delivery, a lesion that is bleeding should be curetted and cauterized (Figure 2.1).

## Changes in the oral mucosa

Pregnancy can exacerbate a pre-existing chronic gingivitis[4] that is usually the result of poor oral hygiene. Histologically, the most prominent change in pregnancy gingivitis is proliferation of capillaries. Clinically, the gingival papillae become enlarged and purple in colour and bleed easily after trauma (Figure 2.2). Stagnation and secondary infection may occur, leading to halitosis. Treatment consists of strict oral hygiene.

Occasionally, a single papilla becomes enlarged to form an epulis, which is a soft tissue swelling of the gingival margin (Figure 2.3). This lesion is sometimes known as the 'pregnancy tumour', but this term

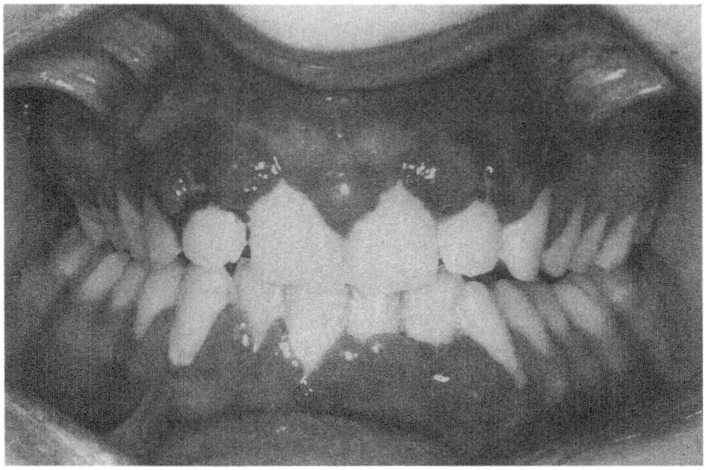

FIGURE 2.2 Pregnancy gingivitis. (Mr D. G. Hillam, Liverpool Dental Hospital)

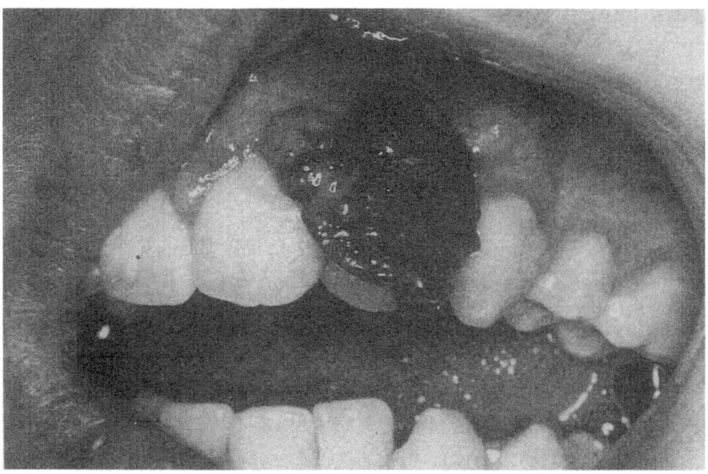

FIGURE 2.3 Pregnancy granuloma. (Mr D. G. Hillam, Liverpool Dental Hospital)

is a misnomer as it is not a neoplasm. The term pregnancy granuloma is preferred because of its histological resemblance to a pyogenic granuloma. It presents in pregnancy as a smooth, soft or semifirm mass. Although some regression is expected after delivery, this may not be complete and the lesion may eventually need to be excised.

## Changes in the hair

Many women comment that their hair seems particularly attractive during pregnancy[5]. This is partly due to the increased percentage of anagen hairs in the second half of pregnancy, leading to decreased shedding. Hormones are known to influence the hair cycle and this effect may be due to the prolongation of the anagen phase by oestrogen.

After delivery, the anagen hairs rapidly enter catagen and then telogen leading to excess shedding. This phenomenon is known as telogen effluvium. It probably occurs to some degree in all women after childbirth but is usually subclinical. In severe cases, diffuse alopecia occurs 1–4 months after delivery. Patients can be reassured that there is usually complete recovery, although this may take up to 15 months to occur.

Women often become more hirsute during pregnancy. This is usually most pronounced on the face but may also involve the limbs and back. It is more common in women who are already constitutionally hirsute. Although there may be some resolution after delivery, it usually persists. If severe hirsutism and virilization occur for the first time during pregnancy, it is important to exclude an underlying cause such as polycystic ovary disease.

## Striae distensae

Striae develop in most women during the second half of pregnancy and there is a familial tendency. They are particularly common in obese women and those carrying large babies. There is still considerable debate about their aetiology. It is generally thought that they are due to the combination of mechanical stretching plus excess adrenocortical hormones. However, Shuster's hypothesis[6] is that they may be solely due to the effect of stretching young adult skin in which the connective tissue is partially mature. He makes the interesting observation that if elderly mature skin is stretched, the skin tears rather than forms striae.

The striae are pink or violaceous and develop opposite to skin tension lines (Figure 2.4). Although they initially occur on the abdomen, they can also develop on the breasts, upper arms, back, thighs, buttocks and inguinal areas. In spite of many home remedies, there is no effective treatment, although reassurance can be given that they will fade with time.

## Pruritus gravidarum

Seventeen per cent of pregnant women itch if all causes of pruritus are taken into account. Pruritus gravidarum is the term used for the small group of women who have itchy but clinically normal skin[7]. In most of these cases the cause remains obscure, but some will have evidence of cholestasis. Cholestasis of pregnancy is thought to be mainly the result of oestrogens interfering with the excretion of bile acids. It is therefore important to check the liver function tests in cases of pruritus gravidarum, particularly if itching is severe.

The abdominal wall is usually the first site to be affected, but itching

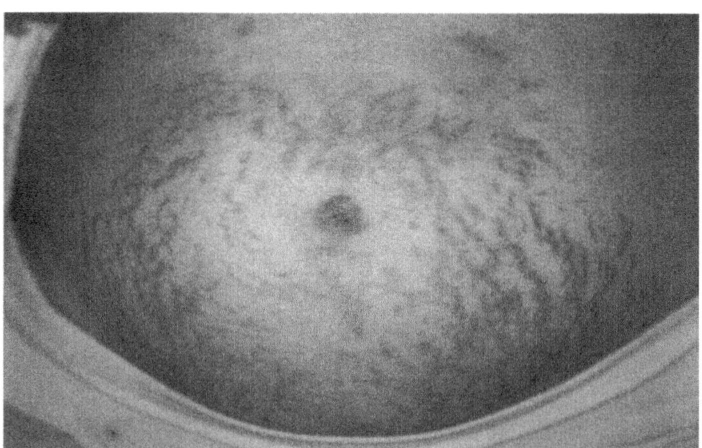

FIGURE 2.4 Striae distensae

may become generalized. It tends to present in the third trimester and to resolve postpartum. Recurrence may occur in further pregnancies or with the use of oral contraceptives.

A topical antipruritic agent such as crotamiton 10% and an oral antihistamine offer symptomatic relief. Although many of the commonly used antihistamines are thought to be safe in pregnancy, it is best only to prescribe a well-established drug such as chlorpheniramine. Brompheniramine should be avoided because it is thought to have teratogenic potential. Cholestyramine, an ion-exchange resin, has been used in severe cases of cholestasis, but it has not been established that it is safe in pregnancy.

## THE EFFECT OF PREGNANCY ON SKIN DISORDERS

Pregnancy has an unpredictable effect on many skin disorders. Some of the most important diseases to be influenced by pregnancy are listed in Table 2.1.

TABLE 2.1 Skin diseases influenced by pregnancy

| *Tendency to improve* | *Variable effect* | *Tendency to deteriorate* |
|---|---|---|
| Atopic eczema | Acne | Pityriasis rosea |
| Psoriasis | Malignant melanoma | Erythema nodosum |
| Alopecia areata | | Candidosis |
| Sarcoidosis | | Condylomata acuminata |
| | | Ehlers–Danlos syndrome |
| | | Neurofibromatosis |
| | | Systemic lupus erythematosus |
| | | Pustular psoriasis |

Modified from Winton, G. B. and Lewis, C. W. (1982). Dermatoses of pregnancy. *J. Am. Acad. Dermatol.*, **6**, 977–98.

## Skin diseases with a tendency to improve in pregnancy

Although controversial, it is thought that pregnancy often has a beneficial effect on atopic eczema. If a mother has atopic eczema, a current theory is that exclusive breast feeding will delay the appearance of atopic eczema in her baby. It has been suggested that this is because the breast-fed baby is exposed to fewer food antigens.

There is thought to be a definite tendency towards improvement or remission of psoriasis during pregnancy, although there is little up-to-date data concerning this. In a study of the natural history of psoriasis by Farber and Nall[8], 32% of women reported an improvement of psoriasis during pregnancy. Pustular psoriasis, however, can be triggered by pregnancy and will be discussed in a later section. Pregnancy can result in the regrowth of hair lost in alopecia areata, but this recovery is usually temporary. Sarcoidosis can also improve, possibly related to the increased levels of corticosteroids in the blood during pregnancy.

## Skin diseases on which pregnancy has a variable effect

### *Acne*

As progesterone and oestrogen have both pro- and anti-inflammatory actions, it is not surprising that the effect of pregnancy on acne is so variable. There are reports showing an improvement in acne during pregnancy and others showing a deterioration[9]. It is absolutely essential that women who are on isotretinoin for acne use an effective method of contraception whilst on this drug and for at least one month after the course has completed, because the drug is a potent teratogen. Tetracycline compounds are also contra-indicated in pregnancy because of their possible adverse effects on the developing bones and teeth of the fetus.

### *Malignant melanoma*

It has been estimated that one third of pregnant women report some change of their pigmented naevi. They can become darker and enlarge, presumably due to the same phenomenon that causes hyperpigmentation in pregnancy. It therefore can be difficult to diagnose malignant melanoma in this setting. Foucar *et al.*[10] reviewed the histology of 128 naevocellular naevi from 86 pregnant patients. None of these naevi had sufficient atypia to suggest a malignant diagnosis. On the basis of their findings, the authors concluded that they would be reluctant to attribute prominent atypia in a melanocytic lesion to 'pregnancy effect'.

The emotive subject of the effect of pregnancy on malignant melanoma continues to be highly controversial. Many reports have stated the adverse effects of pregnancy on melanoma. However, one paper by Holly[11] reviews 11 published studies that quantified an association between pregnancy and melanoma. In 10 of these studies, the adverse effect of pregnancy on survival from melanoma could not be demonstrated. It therefore should not be necessary to terminate the pregnancy if a woman subsequently develops a primary malignant melanoma in that pregnancy. The melanoma should be excised in the usual way with an adequate margin of skin depending on the Breslow thickness.

If a woman develops primary melanoma during pregnancy, it is probably wise to advise her against future pregnancies. This is because the tumour may be in part hormonally stimulated and further hormonal stimulation could reactivate latent metastasis. However, there is no indication to avoid pregnancy because a woman has a past history of malignant melanoma. Prior melanoma does not appear to become reactivated in a subsequent pregnancy and the prognosis will be directly related to the thickness of the tumour (R. M. MacKie, personal communication).

## Skin diseases with a tendency to deteriorate in pregnancy

Many skin conditions can deteriorate during pregnancy (Table 2.1). The eruption of pityriasis rosea can be more severe if it occurs in pregnancy. Pregnancy can act as a stimulus for the development of erythema nodosum. Salvatore and Lynch[12] describe 5 women, all of whom had two or more episodes of erythema nodosum at a time of hormonal change. In each case, pregnancy acted as one of the trigger factors.

### *The effect of pregnancy on immunity*

Belchetz[13] has stated that pregnancy causes in the immune system a 'powerful and long-lasting but ill-understood mayhem'. It seems that there is a selective depression of cell-mediated immunity in pregnancy. This is probably due to a number of causes[14]. Most of the steroid hormones that are elevated in pregnancy are able to depress some aspect of cell-mediated immunity. Human chorionic gonadotrophin may contribute to the immunosuppression. Moreover, there appears to be a decrease in the number of T helper cells causing an imbalance in the T helper to T suppressor cell ratio. In contrast, B cells are apparently unaffected.

These changes allow certain infections to be more severe if they occur during pregnancy. Vaginal candidosis occurs more commonly during pregnancy. This is supported by the fact that vaginal carriage of yeasts occurs twice as frequently in pregnant women[14].

Viral infections will be particularly affected by the depression in cell-mediated immunity. It is possible that pregnancy can lead to the development of the acquired immunodeficiency syndrome in a woman who is positive for the human immunodeficiency virus.

Condylomata acuminata (genital warts) can grow rapidly during pregnancy into large masses that rarely can obstruct vaginal delivery. Another complication is the development of laryngeal warts in the newborn infant owing to transmission of the virus. It is therefore preferable that genital warts are treated prior to delivery. Topical podophyllin should never be used in pregnancy because of its potential toxicity. Chamberlain *et al.*[15] describe an 18-year-old woman who developed severe peripheral neuropathy and delivered a stillborn infant after the application of 25% podophyllum resin to florid vulval warts. Suitable methods of treatment include cryotherapy and the carbon-dioxide laser.

### *Ehlers–Danlos syndrome*

Ehlers–Danlos syndrome is a rare connective tissue disorder that is clinically and genetically heterogeneous. Women with types I and IV Ehlers–Danlos syndrome are at risk of developing serious complications of pregnancy.

*Type I disease*. The clinical features of type I disease include markedly extensible skin, hypermobile joints and a tendency to bruise easily. The skin is very fragile, easily tearing and healing to form thin, atrophic, paper-tissue scars, particularly over bony prominences. The texture may be very soft and has been described like chamois leather skin. It is interesting that these patients usually do not develop striae distensae during pregnancy. Pregnancy complications include severe perineal tears and pelvic prolapse.

*Type IV disease*. Type IV Ehlers–Danlos syndrome has characteristic clinical and biochemical features. The skin is thin and the superficial veins appear prominent. Facial features include large eyes, a peaked nose and thin lips. The diagnosis can be confirmed by demonstrating decreased production of type III collagen by fibroblasts in culture. Type IV disease is associated with very serious pregnancy complications, such as rupture of the aorta or uterus and severe postpartum haemorrhage. A study of the pregnancy complications in type IV Ehlers–Danlos syndrome by Rudd *et al.*[16] estimated that the overall risk of death in each pregnancy was 25%.

It is therefore essential that women with Ehlers–Danlos syndrome are typed so that the high-risk groups can be identified. These patients should be carefully counselled and the risks of pregnancy should be explained. Should pregnancy occur, there is no real preference for either vaginal delivery or elective caesarean section. Both methods of delivery have associated complications and the decision will depend upon local resources.

### *Neurofibromatosis*

The lesions of neurofibromatosis (von Recklinghausen's disease) can progress rapidly during pregnancy, with complete or partial remission in the postpartum period. Lesions of neurofibromatosis that appeared for the first time in pregnancy have been termed fibroma molluscum gravidarum. Swapp and Main[17] reported 19 pregnancies in 10 patients with neurofibromatosis. They found that in all cases both pigmented and nodular lesions increased in size and number during pregnancy. In 7 patients, considerable regression of the nodular lesions occurred following delivery.

### *Systemic lupus erythematosus*

Systemic lupus erythematosus is a disease that mainly affects women during their reproductive age. The effect of pregnancy on systemic lupus erythematosus is controversial. Many reports in the past have stated that pregnancy causes an exacerbation of the disease, particularly in the postpartum period. The postpartum flare is thought to result from the loss of the immunosuppressive effects of progesterone and corticosteroids. However, more recent reports have failed to demonstrate this flare. Lockshin *et al.*[18] carried out a prospective study of 33 pregnancies in 28 women with systemic lupus erythematosus. They matched these patients with a similar group of non-pregnant women. Their results failed to show a higher risk of exacerbation of disease during or after pregnancy. These conflicting reports may be explained by an improvement in the management of systemic lupus erythematosus. In anticipation of any flare, the delivery and postpartum period is often covered by an increased dose of systemic steroids.

It is agreed that systemic lupus erythematosus has a deleterious effect on pregnancy. An increased incidence of prematurity and abortions results in a high fetal loss.

*Lupus anticoagulant*. Pregnant women with systemic lupus erythematosus should be screened for the presence of lupus anticoagulant, which is an acquired antiphospholipid antibody. It is found in 5–15% of women with systemic lupus erythematosus. It is associated with thrombotic episodes, intrauterine death and recurrent spontaneous abortions. High levels of anticardiolipin antibodies are invariably found and their presence acts as a sensitive screening test for the lupus anticoagulant. The activated partial thromboplastin time is usually prolonged. Cutaneous markers include erythematous macules on the fingertips, widespread cutaneous necrosis and leg ulcers[19]. It is important that these women are identified as the risk of abortion may be reduced by early treatment with prednisone and aspirin.

*Neonatal lupus.* The presence of maternal antibodies to SS-A (Ro) antigen acts as a serological marker for neonatal lupus[20], which is a very rare disease. These antibodies are transferred transplacentally and can usually be detected in the sera of affected infants until approximately 6 months of age. Clinical findings in the neonatal lupus syndrome include skin lesions resembling adult discoid lupus and congenital heart block. The skin lesions are usually sun-induced and in most cases they have disappeared by the age of 6 months, correlating with the loss of autoantibodies. In contrast, the heart block is persistent. It is important that these children are followed up, as there have been reports of infants with neonatal lupus developing systemic lupus erythematosus in later life.

*Treatment.* Treatment of systemic lupus erythematosus should not be withheld because the patient is pregnant. If the woman requires systemic prednisolone, the fetus is probably protected by placental II $\beta$-dehydrogenase, which oxidizes the steroid to an inactive form. Dexamethasone, however, should be avoided in pregnancy as it undergoes very limited metabolism by the placenta. The antimalarial drugs, chloroquine and hydroxychloroquine, should not be given in pregnancy because of the possibility of retinal damage to the fetus. The long-term effects of intrauterine exposure to azathioprine are not known. It is thought, however, that azathioprine is probably safe to use in pregnancy, as it is effectively degraded by placental enzymes.

### *Pustular psoriasis of pregnancy (impetigo herpetiformis)*

In 1872, Hebra described an acute pustular eruption, known as impetigo herpetiformis, that occurred in pregnant women. This was thought to be a specific dermatosis of pregnancy and many workers still believe that it is a distinct entity. However, a similar eruption has occurred in non-pregnant women and in men. It is therefore preferable to regard impetigo herpetiformis as a rare variant of pustular psoriasis that is precipitated by pregnancy. Affected women usually have neither personal nor family history of psoriasis.

The histological findings are those of pustular psoriasis, with the presence of Kogoj's spongiform pustules in the epidermis. Pierard *et al.*[21] studied the biopsies from 5 women who had impetigo herpetiformis. They found many large mononuclear cells in the epidermal pustules and in the dermis that are not normally a feature of pustular psoriasis. Patients should be investigated for hypocalcaemia, which has often been reported in this disease.

Pustular psoriasis of pregnancy usually presents during the last 3 months of gestation but can occur as early as the first trimester. The patient may be critically ill with pyrexia, delirium, diarrhoea, vomiting and tetany[7]. Death can occur secondary to cardiac or renal failure. The skin eruption is characteristically symmetrical and involves the flexures. Erythematous patches develop superficial pustules at their margins. The lesions spread peripherally, with the development of crusts in the central areas and moist vegetating plaques may occur in the flexures. The disease can become widespread, although the face, hands and feet are usually spared. The mucous membranes may be involved. The condition tends to remit after delivery, but characteristically recurs, and patients should therefore be advised against further pregnancies. Placental insufficiency can lead to still birth and neonatal death.

The patient must be admitted into hospital and treated as an acute medical emergency. Dehydration, electrolyte imbalance and hypocalcaemia must be corrected. Methotrexate, etretinate and PUVA are contra-indicated in pregnancy. Therefore, if the disease is severe, systemic corticosteroids are the treatment of choice starting at a dose of prednisolone 15–30 mg per day. An antibiotic should also be given if there is evidence of secondary bacterial infection. If the disease continues to deteriorate, termination of pregnancy may be indicated. After delivery, if the disease remains active, methotrexate or etretinate plus PUVA (RePUVA) may be required to act as a steroid sparing agent.

## SPECIFIC DERMATOSES OF PREGNANCY

The list of skin disorders specifically related to pregnancy and the puerperium used to be long and the terminology bewildering. In 1968, Nurse[22] divided the non-bullous pregnancy eruptions into two groups. In the early type, the skin lesions occurred mainly on the limbs and upper trunk. In the late type, the lesions usually affected the abdomen and were often localized to the striae. In 1982, Holmes and Black[23] simplified the classification of the pregnancy dermatoses (Table 2.2). Pregnancy prurigo and polymorphic eruption of pregnancy correlate respectively with the early and late types of eruption described by Nurse.

TABLE 2.2 Classification of the specific dermatoses of pregnancy

| *Old* | *New* |
|---|---|
| Herpes gestationis | Pemphigoid gestationis |
| Early type (Nurse)<br>Early onset prurigo of pregnancy<br>Prurigo gestationis of Besnier<br>Papular dermatitis of pregnancy | Pregnancy prurigo |
| Late type (Nurse)<br>Late onset prurigo of pregnancy<br>Toxaemic rash of pregnancy<br>PUPPP syndrome (pruritic urticarial papules and plaques of pregnancy) | Polymorphic eruption of pregnancy |
| | Pruritic folliculitis of pregnancy |

Modified from Holmes, R. C. and Black, M. M. (1982). The specific dermatoses of pregnancy: a reappraisal with special emphasis on a proposed simplified clinical classification. *Clin. Exp. Dermatol.*, **7**, 65–73.

## Pemphigoid gestationis

This is a rare, autoimmune, vesiculobullous disease of pregnancy that is usually recurrent. The reported incidence ranges widely from 1:3000 to 1:60 000 pregnancies. The misleading term, herpes gestationis, has been replaced by pemphigoid gestationis, because of the clinical and pathological resemblance of the disease to bullous pemphigoid.

### *Aetiology*

Much more is known about the aetiology of pemphigoid gestationis, compared with the other specific dermatoses of pregnancy. Pemphigoid gestationis tends to affect women who are high immune responders. These patients also have a higher incidence of other autoimmune disorders such as Graves' disease. Holmes *et al.*[24], in a study of 25 women with pemphigoid gestationis, found a significant increase in the frequency of the HLA antigen $DR_3$. They also found an increase in the frequency with which $DR_3$ occurred in combination with $DR_4$. Both these antigens can increase the susceptibility of an individual to immunological disease.

A complement binding immunoglobulin G (IgG), known as pemphigoid gestationis factor, is invariably present in the serum of patients with pemphigoid gestationis. The titres of this factor do not correlate with the severity of the disease. The pemphigoid gestationis factor is present in such low levels that it cannot always be detected by routine indirect immunofluorescence techniques. Complement indirect immunofluorescence must be used to demonstrate the pemphigoid gestationis factor. Ortonne *et al.*[25] suggest that the antigenic trigger for this antibody is the basement membrane zone of extra-villous cytotrophoblasts. The placental origin of the antigen is supported by the fact that pemphigoid gestationis can also occur in association with choriocarcinoma and hydatidiform mole. Owing to the antigenic similarity between the amniotic basement membrane zone and the dermo-epidermal junction, the antibody cross-reacts with the skin to form subepidermal bullae in the mother and rarely in the neonate.

The sexual consort may be important in the aetiology of pemphigoid gestationis[24]. Both in pregnancy and the trophoblastic tumours, the woman is exposed to foreign antigens derived from her sexual partner. Some women with a past history of unaffected pregnancies only develop pemphigoid gestationis when they change their partner.

### *Hormonal modulation*

Hormones can exert a modulating effect on pemphigoid gestationis[24]. Oestrogens appear to exacerbate the disease and progestogens may have an immunosuppressive effect. Therefore, a flare of the disease can occur during ovulation or if a patient is subsequently prescribed an oestrogen-containing oral contraceptive pill. Pemphigoid gestationis often remits in the last few weeks of pregnancy, when progesterone levels are high. The fall in progesterone that occurs postpartum can cause a severe exacerbation of the disease. A fall in the level of progesterone may also explain the flare of pemphigoid gestationis that can occur premenstrually.

### *Histology*

The diagnosis of pemphigoid gestationis should always be confirmed by biopsy of a lesion and immunofluorescence of normal perilesional skin. Histology of an urticarial lesion shows epidermal and upper dermal oedema, with a mixed perivascular infiltrate containing eosinophils. Histology of a blister shows a subepidermal bulla, which may contain numerous eosinophils. The subepidermal separation is due to necrosis of basal cells, the earliest change appearing to be damage to the basal cell plasma membrane. Direct immunofluorescence of perilesional skin should show a band-like deposition of C3 at the basement membrane. IgG is demonstrated less frequently. Immunoelectron microscopy reveals that, as in bullous pemphigoid, the C3 deposition occurs within the lamina lucida of the basement membrane.

*Clinical features*

Pemphigoid gestationis presents most frequently in the second trimester. However, it can occur as early as the second week of pregnancy and as late as the early postpartum period. Early lesions consist of itchy, urticated, erythematous papules. These often initially involve the periumbilical region and abdomen before becoming more widespread over the trunk and limbs. The palms and soles can be involved, which may lead to the mistaken diagnosis of scabies. Involvement of the face or mucosae is uncommon. The lesions often have a target-like or geographical configuration and vesicles and tense blisters usually occur over the following days or weeks (Figure 2.5). Pemphigoid gestationis is the only specific dermatosis of pregnancy in which bullae occur. Although the disease generally remits within three months of delivery,

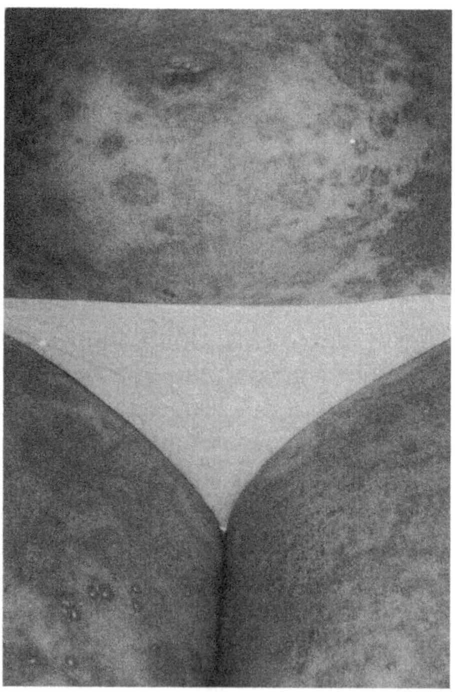

FIGURE 2.5 Pemphigoid gestationis showing target-like lesions and bullae on the right thigh

the course may be protracted, lasting many years. Figure 2.6 shows a patient with widespread lesions of pemphigoid gestationis persisting 6 months after delivery.

There have been conflicting reports about the effect of pemphigoid gestationis on the fetus. Shornick *et al.*[26] failed to show an increased fetal morbidity or mortality in their study of 28 patients with pemphigoid gestationis. Holmes and Black[27], however, studied the infants of 50 affected pregnancies and found an increased incidence of infants that were 'small for dates'. This finding could be related to placental dysfunction. As such infants may have an increased mortality and morbidity, Holmes and Black suggest that it is necessary that women with pemphigoid gestationis are delivered in units where facilities are available for intensive care of the newborn. The incidence of bullous lesions in these infants is very uncommon, which is surprising as the maternal anti-basement membrane zone antibody is thought to cross the placenta.

Pemphigoid gestationis tends to recur in subsequent pregnancies although unaffected or 'skipped' pregnancies can occur. Recurrences may present at an earlier stage in pregnancy and be more severe. The disease is therefore a relative contra-indication to further pregnancies. The potential risks of recurrent pemphigoid gestationis should be made clear to any woman with a history of the disease. These women should not be prescribed the oestrogen-containing oral contraceptive pill, as this may cause an exacerbation of the disease. The progesterone-only pill, however, may be tolerated.

### *Treatment*

A mild case of pemphigoid gestationis can be treated symptomatically, with a topical corticosteroid and an oral antihistamine, such as chlorpheniramine. If bullae occur, a course of oral prednisolone should be given, starting at 40 mg per day. Once the disease is under control, the dose can be reduced to a lower maintenance level. The steroid requirement often falls in the last few weeks of gestation but a postpartum flare should be anticipated by a corresponding increase in the dose of prednisolone. The prednisolone should be discontinued when the disease finally goes into remission.

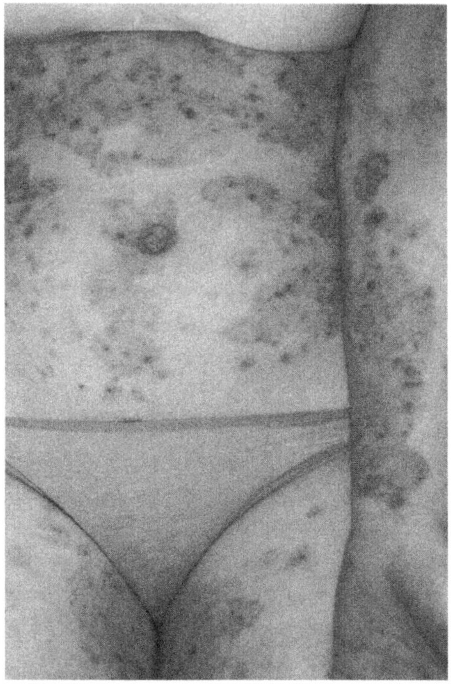

FIGURE 2.6 Pemphigoid gestationis persisting 6 months after delivery. (Patient of Dr M. M. Molokhia)

## Pregnancy prurigo

This is a non-bullous specific dermatosis of pregnancy of unknown aetiology. The reported incidence ranges from 1:50 to 1:300 pregnancies. Nurse[22] found that the incidence of pregnancy prurigo was three times that of polymorphic eruption of pregnancy.

The diagnosis of pregnancy prurigo is based on the clinical findings. It usually presents between the 25th and 29th weeks of gestation. Itchy, excoriated, grouped papules develop on the extensor surfaces of the limbs and upper trunk and secondary eczematous changes can occur. Resolution usually occurs after delivery, often leaving postinflammatory hypermelanosis. Occasionally, lesions can persist for up to 3 months postpartum. The disease does not tend to recur in subsequent pregnancies and the fetal prognosis is thought to be unaffected.

Spangler *et al.*[28] described a disease that was termed papular dermatitis of pregnancy. In their cases, crusted, papular lesions were widely scattered over the body. Holmes and Black[23] suggest that these cases were severe examples of pregnancy prurigo. Spangler found an associated high fetal mortality rate of 27%, but careful analysis of the data[7,23] suggests that this is an overestimate, and this finding has not been confirmed by other workers.

Treatment is symptomatic and a systemic corticosteroid is not required.

## Polymorphic eruption of pregnancy

Polymorphic eruption of pregnancy is thought to be the commonest of the specific pregnancy dermatoses. The reported incidence ranges from 1:120 to 1:240 pregnancies. It is a distinct clinical entity of unknown aetiology.

The diagnosis of polymorphic eruption of pregnancy is based on the clinical presentation. Histological findings are non-specific and include epidermal and upper dermal oedema with a perivascular lymphohistiocytic infiltrate that often contains eosinophils. Established lesions may show vesicular spongiosis, but subepidermal bullae are absent and direct and indirect immunofluorescence is negative. These findings help to differentiate this disease from pemphigoid gestationis.

Polymorphic eruption of pregnancy has a predilection for primigravidae and usually presents late in the third trimester. The average time of onset is the 35th week of gestation. Early lesions consist of erythematous papules that coalesce to form urticarial plaques. Occasionally, tiny vesicles and target lesions occur. Lesions invariably begin on the abdomen, often in association with prominent striae. They may spread to involve the thighs, buttocks and limbs (Figure 2.7). The periumbilical region is usually spared, which helps to distinguish polymorphic eruption of pregnancy from the early stage of pemphigoid gestationis[29]. Although the rash tends to be extremely itchy, excoriations are seldom found. The duration of the eruption is usually 6 weeks and resolution can be expected within 2 weeks postpartum.

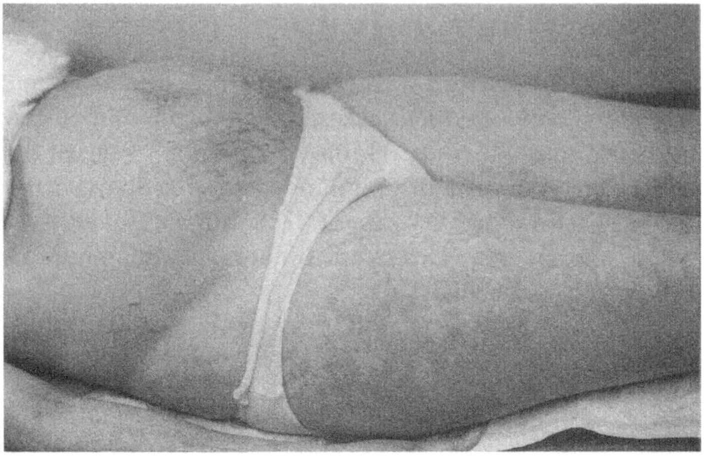

FIGURE 2.7 Polymorphic eruption of pregnancy showing prominent striae and urticarial lesions over the thighs

Polymorphic eruption of pregnancy is not associated with any maternal or fetal complications and it does not tend to recur in subsequent pregnancies.

Symptomatic relief can usually be obtained with a topical corticosteroid and an oral antihistamine. There should be no need for a systemic corticosteroid.

## Pruritic folliculitis of pregnancy

This term was suggested by Zoberman and Farmer[30] after they had studied a pruritic, erythematous, papular eruption occurring in 6 pregnant women. In 5 of the 6 cases, an acute folliculitis was seen on histological examinations. Microorganisms were not found and the aetiology is unknown.

The condition presents between the 4th and 9th months of gestation. The lesions are usually widespread and consist of small, excoriated, erythematous papules. Resolution can be expected by 1 month post-partum. The fetal prognosis is unaffected but the disease may recur in subsequent pregnancies. No particular treatment has been found to be effective.

## REFERENCES


1. Wong, R. C. and Ellis, C. N. (1984). Physiologic skin changes in pregnancy. *J. Am. Acad. Dermatol.*, **10,** 929–940
2. Sanchez, N. P., Pathak, M. A., Sato, S., Fitzpatrick, T. B., Sanchez, J. L. and Mihm, M. C. (1981). Melasma: A clinical, light microscopic, ultrastructural and immunofluorescence study. *J. Am. Acad. Dermatol.*, **4,** 698–710
3. Vázquez, M., Ibañez, M. I. and Sánchez, J. L. (1986). Pigmentary demarcation lines during pregnancy. *Cutis*, **38,** 263–266
4. Tyldesley, W. R. (1981). The oral mucosa in generalised disease. In *Oral Medicine*, pp. 138–139. (Oxford: Oxford University Press)
5. Rook, A. and Dawber, R. (1982). Diffuse alopecia. In *Diseases of the Hair and Scalp*, pp. 123–124. (Oxford: Blackwell Scientific)
6. Shuster, S. (1979). The cause of striae distensae. *Acta Dermatol. Venereol.* (*Stockh.*) *Suppl.*, **59,** 161–169
7. Winton, G. G. and Lewis, C. W. (1982). Dermatoses of pregnancy. *J. Am. Acad. Dermatol.*, **6,** 977–998
8. Farber, E. M. and Nall, M. L. (1974). The natural history of psoriasis in 5,600 patients. *Dermatologica*, **148,** 1–18
9. Cunliffe, W. J. and Cotterill, J. A. (1975). Clinical features of the acnes. In *The Acnes*, p. 13. (London: W. B. Saunders)
10. Foucar, E., Bentley, T. J., Laube, D. W. and Rosai, J. (1985). A histopathologic evaluation of nevocellular nevi in pregnancy. *Arch. Dermatol.*, **121,** 350–354
11. Holly, E. A. (1986). Melanoma and pregnancy. *Rec. Results Cancer Res.*, **102,** 118–126
12. Salvatore, M. A. and Lynch, P. J. (1980). Erythema nodosum, estrogens, and pregnancy. *Arch. Dermatol.*, **116,** 557–558
13. Belchetz, P. E. (1987). Thyroid disease in pregnancy. *Br. Med. J.*, **294,** 264–265
14. Weinberg, E. D. (1984). Pregnancy-associated depression of cell-mediated immunity. *Rev. Infect. Dis.*, **6,** 814–830
15. Chamberlain, M. J., Reynolds, A. L. and Yeoman, W. B. (1972). Topical effect of podophyllum application in pregnancy. *Br. Med. J.*, **3,** 391–392
16. Rudd, N. L., Holbrook, K. A., Nimrod, C. and Byers, P. H. (1983). Pregnancy complications in type IV Ehlers–Danlos syndrome. *Lancet*, **1,** 50–53
17. Swapp, G. H. and Main, R. A. (1973). Neurofibromatosis in pregnancy. *Br. J. Dermatol.*, **80,** 431–435
18. Lockshin, M. D., Reinitz, E., Druzin, M. L., Murrman, M. and Estes, D. (1984). Lupus pregnancy. Case-control prospective study demonstrating absence of lupus exacerbation during or after pregnancy. *Am. J. Med.*, **77,** 893–898
19. Grob, J.-J. and Bonerandi, J.-J., (1986). Cutaneous manifestations associated with the presence of the lupus anticoagulant. A report of two cases and a review of the literature. *J. Am. Acad. Dermatol.*, **15,** 211–219
20. Weston, W. L., Harmon, C., Peebles, C., Manchester, D., Franco, H. L., Huff,

J. C. and Norris D. A. (1982). A serological marker for neonatal lupus erythematosus. *Br. J. Dermatol.*, **107**, 377–382

21. Pierard, G. E., Pierard-Franchimont, C. and de la Brassinne, M. (1983). Impetigo herpetiformis and pustular psoriasis during pregnancy. *Am. J. Dermatopathol.*, **5**, 215–220
22. Nurse, D. S. (1968). Prurigo of pregnancy. *Aust. J. Dermatol.*, **9**, 258–267
23. Holmes, R. C. and Black, M. M. (1982). The specific dermatoses of pregnancy: a reappraisal with special emphasis on a proposed simplified clinical classification. *Clin. Exp. Dermatol.*, **7**, 65–73
24. Holmes, R. C., Black, M. M., Jurecka, W., Dann, J., James, D. C. O., Timlin, D. and Bhogal, B. (1983). Clues to the aetiology and pathogenesis of herpes gestationis. *Br. J. Dermatol.*, **109**, 131–139
25. Ortonne, J.-P., Hsi, B. -L., Verrando, P., Bernerd, F., Pautrat, G., Pisani, A. and Yeh, C.-J. G. (1987). Herpes gestationis factor reacts with the amniotic epithelial basement membrane. *Br. J. Dermatol.*, **117**, 147–154
26. Shornick, J. K., Bangert, J. L., Freeman, R. G., and Gilliam, J. N. (1983). Herpes gestationis: Clinical and histologic features of twenty-eight cases. *J. Am. Acad. Dermatol.*, **8**, 214–224
27. Holmes, R. C. and Black, M. M. (1984). The fetal prognosis in pemphigoid gestationis (herpes gestationis). *Br. J. Dermatol.*, **110**, 67–72
28. Spangler, A. S., Reddy, W., Bardawil, W. A., Roby. C. C. and Emerson, K. (1962). Papular dermatitis of pregnancy. *J. Am. Med. Assoc.*, **181**, 577–581
29. Holmes, R. C., Black, M. M., Dann, J., James, D. C. O. and Bhogal, B. (1982). A comparative study of toxic erythema of pregnancy and herpes gestationis. *Br. J. Dermatol.*, **106**, 499–510
30. Zoberman, E. and Farmer, E. R. (1981). Pruritic folliculitis of pregnancy. *Arch. Dermatol.*, **117**, 20–22

# 3

# LICHEN PLANUS

*R. A. C. GRAHAM-BROWN*

## INTRODUCTION

The papular disorder of skin and mucous membranes known as lichen planus (LP) is encountered throughout the world. LP has no particular predilection for any geographical area or racial group apart from the occurrence of light-induced LP (or LP actinicus), which has been reported much more frequently in sunny countries. Women seem to be affected slightly more often than men in most series[1,2], although Samman[3] found exactly the opposite. It is predominantly a disorder of the middle years of life, but it may present for the first time in old age and occasionally occurs in childhood.

In most instances LP is a self-limiting process, although the time-course varies. Two thirds of the cases of LP in the series reported by Altman and Perry[1] resolved with an average duration of 15 months. However, some patients have LP for years and certain clinical forms are particularly prone to run a prolonged time-course. Notable examples of this are hypertrophic LP and erosive or atrophic LP of skin and mucous membranes. There are some patients who suffer more than one episode of LP and occasional familial incidence has also been recorded.

LP is, of course, a familiar sight to the dermatologist and accounts for approximately 1% of new referrals to skin clinics[4]. Because of its tendency to affect mucous membranes, LP also presents to dentists and oral surgeons, genitourinary physicians and gynaecologists. These groups are therefore usually quite familiar with LP and its manifestations. LP is, however, encountered only rarely by family doctors or general physicians. By my calculations, a general practitioner in the United Kingdom would not expect to see a new case of LP more often than approximately once every 5 years. It is therefore not surprising that LP, with its wide variety of clinical features, can cause considerable diagnostic difficulty. As LP may appear in a number of important clinical situations that may bring it first to the attention of the non-dermatologist (see below), it is important that knowledge and understanding of LP should not be limited to a few specialist groups.

## Lichen and lichenoid

Although it is generally agreed that the first description of LP itself was given by Erasmus Wilson in 1869[5], the word *lichen* or *leichen*, from the Greek λειχηνες, has been used for describing skin disease since classical times. When Robert Willan produced his seminal work *On Cutaneous Diseases*[6], he included lichen under the order PAPULAE. He states that 'Amidst so much confusion, it becomes difficult to fix the proper signification of the word Lichen ... I think ... we may establish an useful distinction in Cutaneous Disorders, if, in conformity to the original sense of the word, the Lichen be defined, an extensive eruption of Papulae affecting adults, connected with internal disorder, usually terminating in Scurf; recurrent; not contagious.'

One of the problems that the dermatologist has when he discusses with his general colleagues LP and the other disorders that bear the title *lichen* or *lichenoid(es)* results from our current use of these words. There are now many disorders that have lichen or lichenoid(es) in their title (see Table 3.1), most of which bear no relationship to LP or to each other except for a superficial clinical resemblance that is only marginal in some instances. Furthermore, we have become used to describing any flat-topped papular eruption as lichenoid, and at the same time using lichenoid to describe a particular pathological picture that has features reminiscent of LP. Such histopathological changes (see below) certainly can result in clinical appearances that resemble LP too, but this is not always the case. For example, poikiloderma vasculare atrophicans has a *lichenoid* histology and, although a flat-

TABLE 3.1 Diseases bearing the name *lichen* or *lichenoid(es)*

| | |
|---|---|
| Lichen aureus (purpuricus) | Keratosis lichenoides chronica* |
| Lichen amyloidosus | Parapsoriasis lichenoides |
| Lichen myxoedematosus | Pityriasis lichenoides chronica |
| Lichen nitidus | Pityriasis lichenoides et varioliformis acuta |
| Lichen nuchae | Pigmented purpuric lichenoid dermatosis of Gougerot and Blum |
| Lichen (ruber) planus | Lichenoid sarcoid |
| Lichen sclerosus et atrophicus | Lichenoid syphilide |
| Lichen scrofulosorum | |
| Lichen simplex chronicus | |
| Lichen spinulosa | |
| Lichen striatus | |
| Lichen urticatus | |
| Lichen verrucosus et reticularis* | |

* Synonyms for the same disorder (sometimes known as Nekam's disease)

topped, papular element may be present there is usually no resemblance to LP at all. Furthermore, some of the disorders listed in Table 3.1 have no histopathological features remotely suggestive of LP, while exhibiting a so-called *lichenoid* clinical appearance.

There is much to commend the view of Pinkus[7], who writes of *lichenoid tissue reactions,* where basal cell damage and the consequences of this are the essential features. He points out that such changes are present in a number of disorders with different clinical features. It seems to me that the term *lichenoid* should be reserved for one of its uses: I would prefer to retain *lichenoid* in its pathological context, where it has a more specific meaning[7] and find some other way of describing eruptions that happen to resemble LP clinically. Perhaps the term *LP-like* would be appropriate. In many situations, when a precise diagnosis is not possible on clinical grounds and the resemblance to LP is not very close, it may be more satisfactory to attempt to go no further than to describe the eruption as papular.

## CLINICAL FEATURES OF LICHEN PLANUS AND ITS VARIANTS

LP may appear under various guises, and can affect any part of the body surface, including orificial epithelia, hair and nails. There are several clinical patterns that are generally accepted as variants of LP (see Table 3.2). There is also some debate about others (such as lichen nitidus) that I have included in Table 3.1, but discussion of the possible relationship between these is beyond the scope of this chapter.

### 'Classical' lichen planus

This is the commonest presentation of LP, although in follow-up clinics the more long-lived forms of LP are more frequently encountered. This is because, as has already been mentioned, most cases of LP are self-limiting and the classical form typically resolves in due course. As mentioned above, the time-course is variable but a typical attack lasts for a few months and most have cleared by 18

TABLE 3.2 Clinical variants of lichen planus

| |
|---|
| Classical |
| Actinic |
| Annular |
| Atrophic |
| Bullous |
| Erythrodermic |
| Exanthematic/guttate |
| Hypertrophicus |
| LP/LE overlap |
| Lichen planopilaris (follicular LP) |
| Lichen planus pemphigoides |
| Lichen planus pigmentosus (+erythema dyschromicum perstans?) |
| Linear |
| Micropapular |
| Hands and feet |
| Mucosal |
| Nail |

months. There are many excellent descriptions of LP, most of which emphasize the features that are seen in the typical case, and so I shall not dwell on this aspect. However, we should briefly review the clinical features.

In classical LP, lesions appear without warning, usually on the major sites of predilection: the anterior surface of the wrists, the small of the back and around the lower legs and ankles. Itching is often a prominent complaint and can be unbearably intense but is not always present and its absence should not of itself cause the diagnosis to be revised. The lesions of classical LP are papules that vary in size from a millimetre to a centimetre or so across (Figure 3.1). The traditional descriptive adjectives that are used about LP papules are 'flat-topped', 'shiny', 'polygonal' and 'violaceous'. In fact, the presence or absence of any of these features depends to a considerable extent on the age of the lesion. The lesions begin as small, pink, dome-shaped papules that rapidly expand and take on a flat-topped morphology. Sometimes the lesions have a small central depression. The colour may become

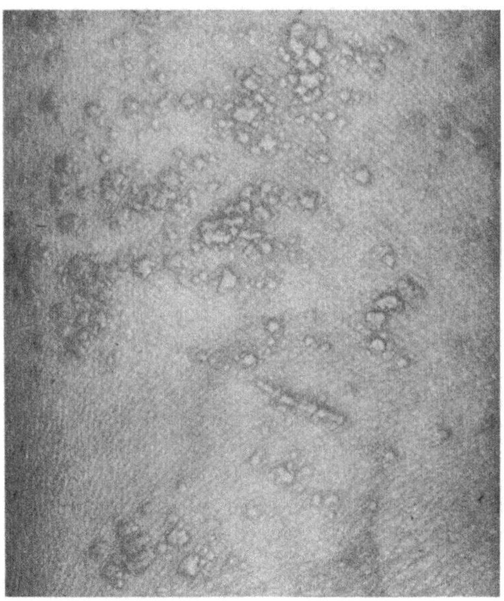

FIGURE 3.1 Typical flat-topped papules on the forearm. A good example of the Köbner phenomenon is also clearly seen

quite a bright red before it finally goes duskier and achieves the purplish-red hue that is traditionally called 'violaceous', which literally means like the colour of the violet family. It is this redness that led Hebra to call the disorder 'lichen ruber'[8]. Indeed, some European authors still call LP 'lichen ruber planus'. The colour of the LP papule is also, of course, affected by the background pigmentation of the skin on which it arises, but it is important to remember that pigmentary incontinence is common and can be very marked. Each papule lasts for a few weeks before resolving, often leaving a patch of pigmentation as its calling-card. Scattered small patches of hyperpigmentation at the site of previous papules are a useful diagnostic sign in LP.

Two other very important features must be mentioned. The first is that LP papules may be surmounted by a fine network of white lines or dots known as Wickham's striae (Figure 3.2). These are pathognomonic of LP. The second is that LP may exhibit the Köbner phenomenon and appear in cuts, scars and scratch-marks (Fig 3.1). Although other disorders, and particularly psoriasis, may show this feature, it can be helpful in distinguishing LP from other papular skin disorders.

Mucosal and, particularly, oral changes are extremely common.

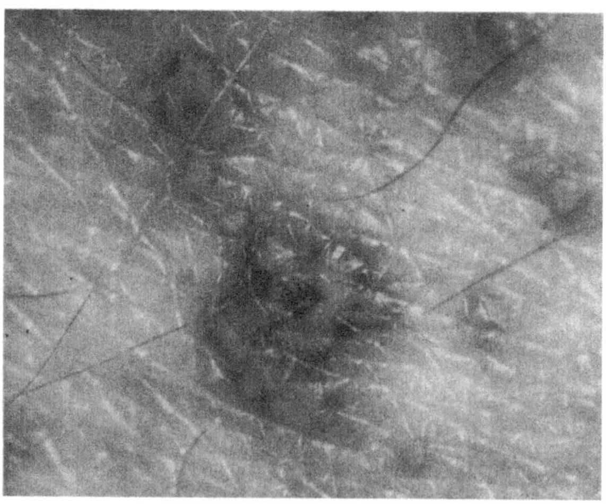

FIGURE 3.2 Wickham's striae: dusky LP papules are surmounted by irregularly shaped paler areas

The reported incidence varies from 30 to 70%. I shall return to the oral lesions of LP later.

## Lichen planus variants

*Actinic* LP is the term used to describe the appearance of LP lesions exclusively (or virtually so) on light-exposed surfaces. There are some who are not convinced that the eruption is always sufficiently characteristic of LP to justify the designation of a distinct LP actinicus variant[9]. However, there are certainly well-documented cases that have had all the features of LP but in which the eruption has been light-provoked[10,11]. Furthermore, it has been possible to reproduce LP lesions with typical histological features by using artificial UV sources[11]. Interestingly, a light-induced LP-like eruption may also be associated with ingestion of drugs, especially the thiazides.

Actinic LP occurs predominantly in dark-skinned individuals and in very sunny countries, but I have seen a case in Britain in a fair-skinned girl with Down's syndrome (Figure 3.3).

*Annular* lesions are not uncommon in LP and are formed by the gradual extension of LP papules with clearing in the centre. This

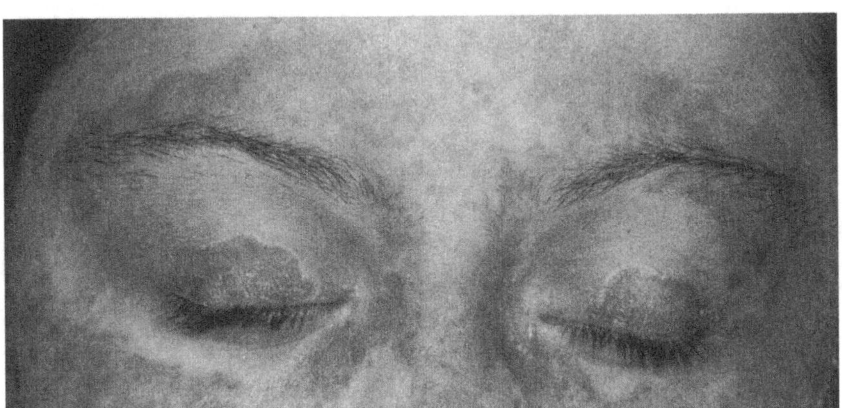

FIGURE 3.3 Actinic LP: there are annular lesions that developed after exposure to sun

central area is often pigmented (Figure 3.4). These ring-forms may occur in the midst of otherwise typical LP or may occur on their own. It is particularly common to see this phenomenon on the penis.

*Atrophic* LP is a troublesome form of the disease. It is rarer on the skin than in the mouth. I shall return to atrophic LP of the mouth in due course. When it occurs on the skin, it often provides diagnostic difficulty and a biopsy is usually required to confirm the diagnosis. Such changes are most commonly seen on the feet, where eroded areas often accompany marked hyperkeratosis of the soles and a dystrophy of the nails.

*Bullous* LP and LP *pemphigoides* are best considered together. The terms are used to describe the appearance of blisters in LP. In bullous LP, dermoepidermal damage is greater than usual and small vesicles and bullae appear within or on pre-existing LP lesions. In LP pemphigoides, the bullae appear on normal skin, and may precede, follow or accompany typical LP papules elsewhere on the skin. The clinical picture in LP pemphigoides is of an acute eruption of bullae and the changes may be sufficiently severe and widespread to resemble dermatitis herpetiformis, bullous pemphigoid or even pemphigus. The

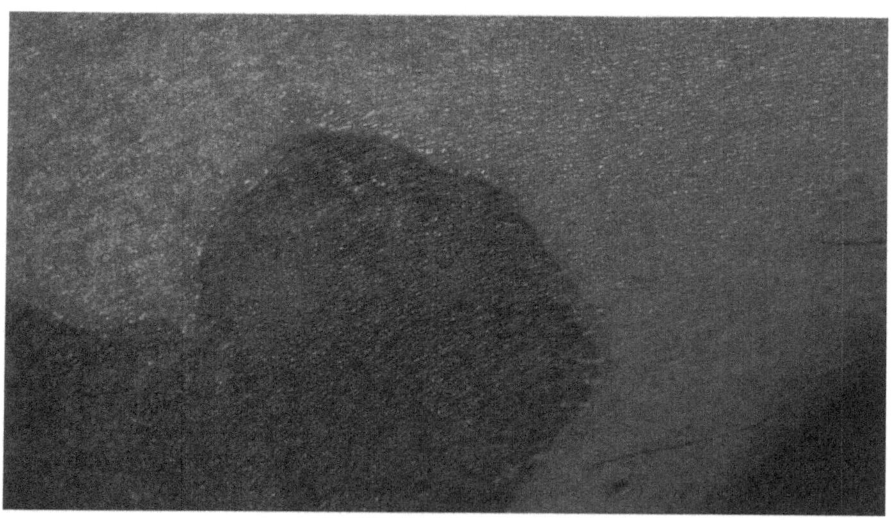

FIGURE 3.4 Annular LP: this lesion on the neck shows marked post-inflammatory hyperpigmentation in the centre

clinical differences between bullous LP and LP pemphigoides are most clearly delineated in a paper by Sarkany and colleagues[12]. The distinction is emphasized by the finding of linear basement membrane zone IgG and C3 in patients labelled as LP pemphigoides[13], although this then gives rise to the debate as to whether this situation is better interpreted as co-existing LP and bullous pemphigoid[14]. However, there may also be a circulating antibody in LP pemphigoides that appears to be distinct from that seen in bullous pemphigoid[14]. One explanation for these curious findings is that LP pemphigoides represents a BP-like immunological response to the tissue damage resulting from LP[15].

*Erythrodermic* LP is very rare and simply represents exceptionally widespread disease.

By *exanthematic* or *guttate* LP is meant an acutely eruptive form of the disease in which the individual lesions usually remain small. The process tends to settle fairly quickly, but the irritation can be appallingly severe, necessitating hospitalization and systemic steroid therapy.

*Hypertrophic* LP is common. Marked hyperkeratotic thickening of the lesions occurs, possibly partly as a result of scratching, 'Köbnerization' and secondary lichenification, because hypertrophic LP is intensely itchy. The usual site is the lower legs (Figure 3.5). The lesions tend to persist for years. There are documented cases of malignant change developing within plaques of hypertrophic LP[16].

The *LP/lupus erythematosus* (*LE*) overlap is a difficult problem[17,18]. Patients in this category have histological and immunofluorescence findings suggestive of LP, while the clinical appearances together with certain laboratory investigations, such as antinuclear antibodies, are more in favour of LE. It is not clear what these patients represent, but it has been suggested that they may imply common pathogenetic mechanisms in both LP and LE[18].

*Lichen planopilaris* or *follicular* LP is the term applied to LP affecting the hair follicle. Although follicular lesions may occur together with typical papular LP, it is more common for them to appear independently. On skin with a low hair density, the eruption is one of spiky projections centred on hair follicles (Figure 3.6). In the scalp, follicular LP may cause an extensive cicatricial alopecia. Nail changes are also commonly seen with this form of LP.

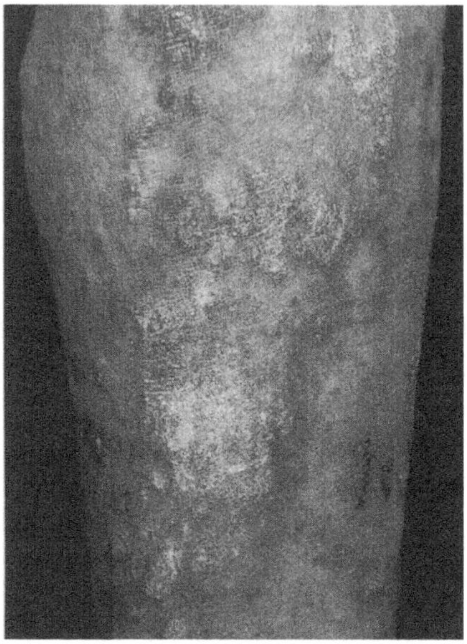

FIGURE 3.5 Hypertrophic LP: typical lesions on the shin

LP *pigmentosus* is the term applied to pigmented patches, usually in Asians, which appear without pre-existing papules, but which show typical histological changes of LP. A good example is shown in Figure 3.7, where the lesions are also slightly atrophic. Rather similar changes have been described in South American patients, where the term *erythema dyschromicum perstans* (ashy dermatosis of Ramirez) is generally applied.

LP is one of several skin diseases that may produce *linear* lesions, which may be associated with LP elsewhere or be the only lesions present. The extent is variable, from a few centimetres to the whole length of a limb.

*Micropapular* LP is a form in which the lesions never enlarge beyond a millimetre or so (Figure 3.8). Differentiation from lichen nitidus may be difficult and some authors feel that there is no real distinction[4]. I do not share this view.

LP of the *hands and feet* can give rise to diagnostic confusion, largely because the typical colour is lost. The papules appear semilucent and often have an umbilication in the centre. A rare form of palmar and,

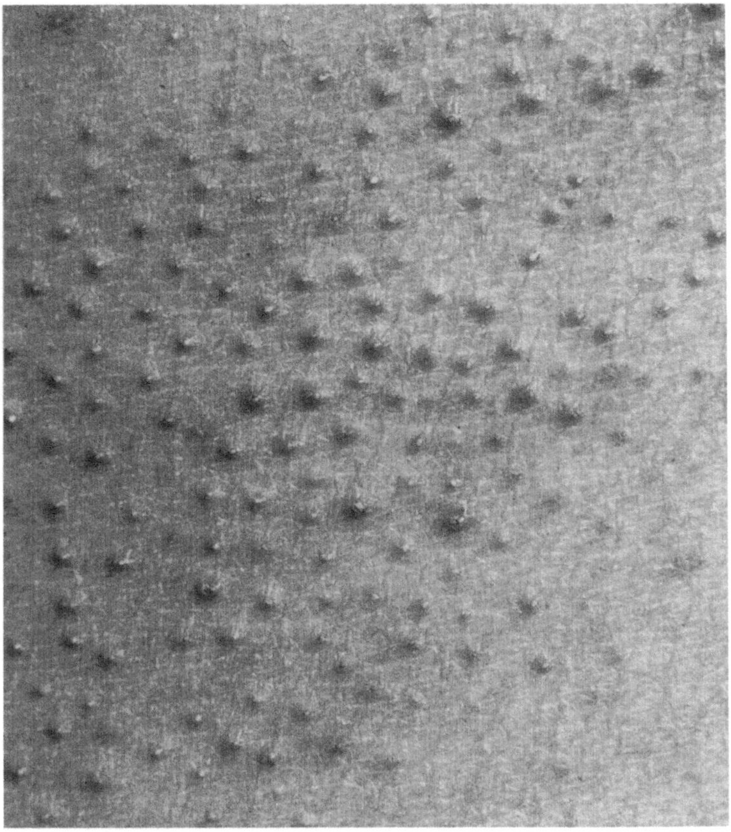

FIGURE 3.6 Lichen planopilaris

particularly, plantar LP has already been mentioned (see atrophic LP above). There is a combination of hyperkeratosis, a marked nail dystrophy and erosive areas.

*Mucosal* LP is very important. LP may affect the mouth, genitalia (in both male and female), anal skin, pharynx and even the oesophagus. The commonest is oral involvement. The changes are most frequently seen on the buccal epithelium, but may occur on the tongue, palate, gingivae and lips[19]. The lesions are most typically a lacy network of lines (Figure 3.9), but there may be a pronounced papular component giving rise to a very rough feel. Occasionally, especially on the tongue, there is a single plaque of LP present. Apart from the

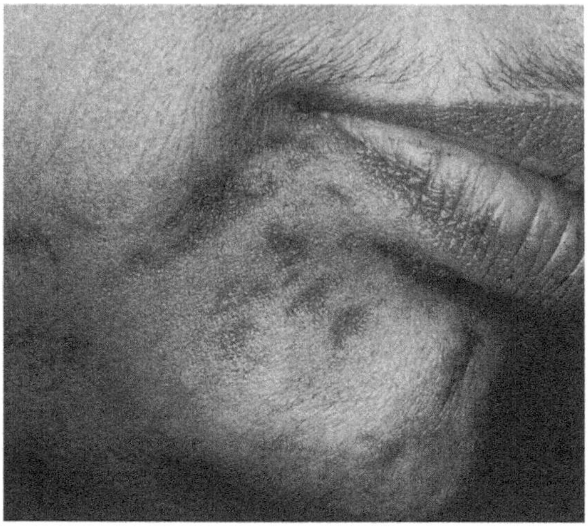

FIGURE 3.7 Lichen planus pigmentosus: histology from one of these areas showed typical LP

feeling of roughness, such lesions are usually asymptomatic. Indeed, many patients only find out that they have oral LP at a routine dental check.

The tongue is also the commonest site for atrophic LP, although other parts of the mouth may be affected. This may be asymmetrical but more often affects the whole of the dorsal surface. The tongue looks flat and shiny and the patient may complain of soreness, especially after eating hot or spicy food. The sensation of taste is often impaired or lost altogether.

The major concern in oral LP is the possible pre-malignant potential. This remains a controversial area. However, although dysplastic changes may certainly be found on biopsy, the risk of carcinoma is probably no more than 2%[20].

*Genital* LP is more common in men than women. Papules on the penis are a common finding in classical LP and annular lesions may also occur. Occasionally, atrophic LP involves the glans and this can be very troublesome. Vulval LP may be difficult to distinguish from lichen sclerosus et atrophicus. Alternatively, there may be nasty inflamed and eroded areas that give rise to a great deal of discomfort.

LP of other mucosal surfaces, such as the anus, pharynx or oeso-

FIGURE 3.8 Micropapular LP

phagus are rare and are usually chance findings.

Nail changes in LP are seen in about 10% of cases[4] but are often overlooked. Early, reversible changes include linear ridges and depressions and a slight thinning of the nail plate. More severe changes, however, may result in complete distortion of the nail (Figure 3.10). The final outcome of severe nail LP is total destruction of the nail apparatus, which may take the form of pterygium. This usually occurs with extensive skin changes, but isolated nail changes, typical of LP, may occur without any other lesions at all. A biopsy of the nail

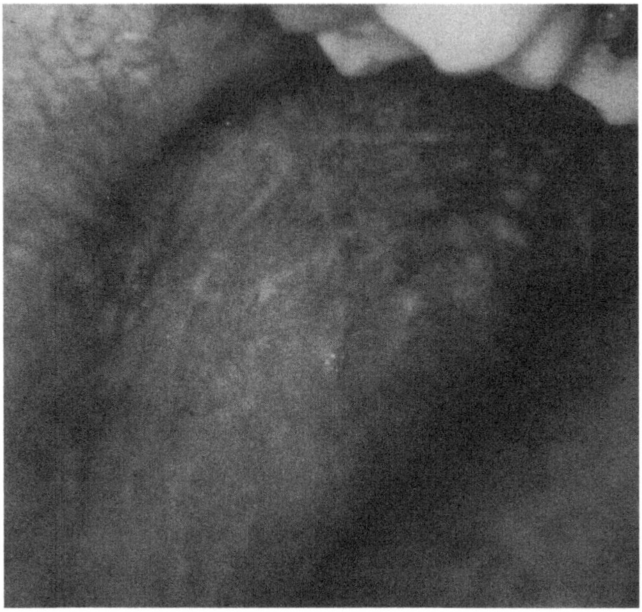

FIGURE 3.9 Oral LP: white lacy lines are visible on the buccal epithelium

or nail fold will reveal the nature of the process if there is diagnostic doubt.

## HISTOPATHOLOGY AND IMMUNOPATHOLOGY OF LICHEN PLANUS

### Histopathology

All these diverse clinical forms are united by a histopathological picture which, when fully developed in a typical papule, is absolutely characteristic (Figure 3.11). There are several essential features.

1. There is a dense, band-like infiltrate in the papillary dermis. This is composed largely of lymphocytes, with some histiocytes. Occasional acute inflammatory cells and plasma cells are also seen. There is extension of this infiltrate into the lower part of the epidermis.

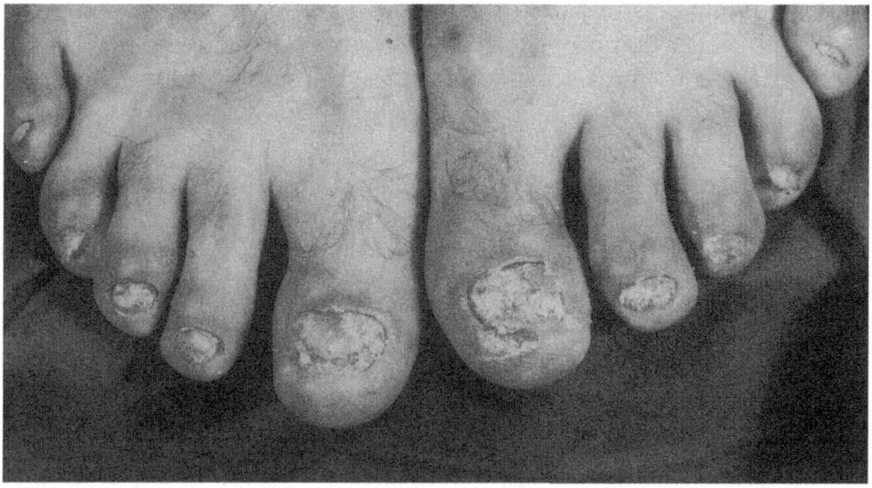

FIGURE 3.10 LP nails: these nails had been treated for months as a fungal infection. A biopsy from the nail-fold confirmed the diagnosis of LP. (I am grateful to Dr I Sarkany for permission to publish this photograph)

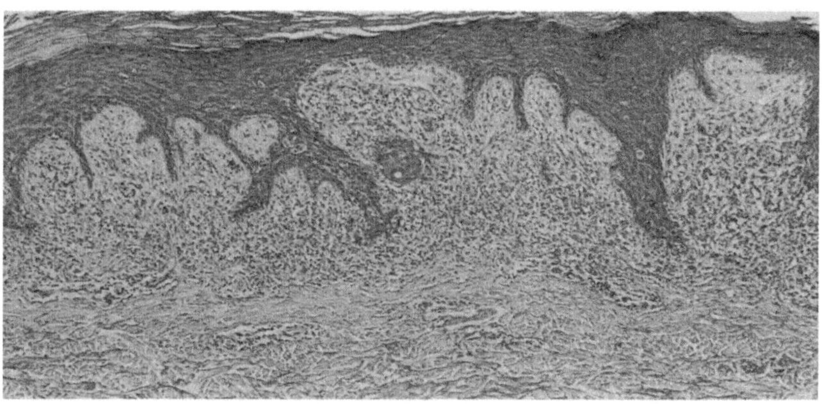

FIGURE 3.11 The histology of LP: there is an upper dermal infiltrate with a 'saw-toothed' pattern to the dermo-epidermal interface.

2. Liquefaction degeneration of the basal layer of the epidermis and the formation of cytoid or *Civatte* bodies (Figure 3.12). Both of these features appear before the dermal infiltrate reaches its full intensity[21,22].
3. The result of processes (1) and (2) is a blurring of the dermo-epidermal junction with the formation of small clefts or *Max Joseph* spaces. The overall effect is often described as a saw-toothed appearance.
4. There is irregular acanthosis and a focal or wedge-shaped increase in the thickness of the granular cell layer (Figure 3.12).

It should be noted that this constellation of histopathological features only occurs in the fully-established papule. LP, like any other disorder, is a dynamic process and the precise changes will be affected by the age of the lesion that is biopsied. For example, in very early lesions the infiltrate is largely perivascular, and mast cells are visible as well as lymphocytes and histiocytes[23]. The earliest significant changes visible within the epidermis are an increase in mononuclear cells many of which are seen on electron microscopy to be Langerhans cells[22] and vacuolar degeneration of the basal keratinocytes. In older lesions, all that may be seen are marked pigmentary changes with the remnants

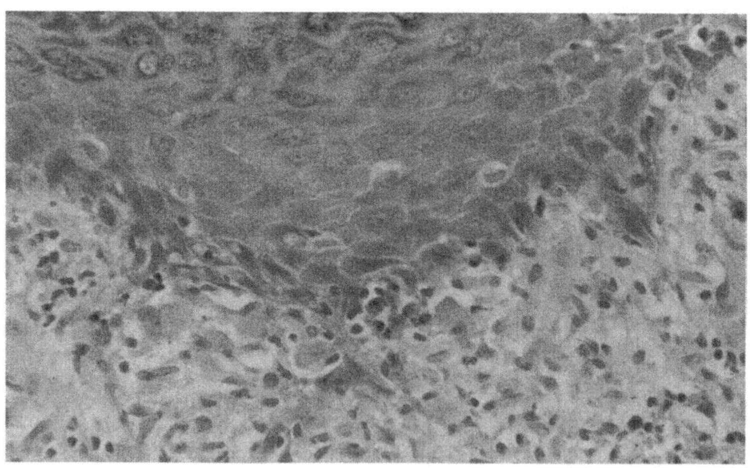

FIGURE 3.12 The histology of LP: granular cell hyperplasia, basal cell degeneration and Civatte body formation are all visible

of an inflammatory infiltrate that contains melanophages. It has also been stressed that fibrosis may occur during the healing phase[23].

There are histological variations in some of the different clinical forms. For example, in atrophic LP the epidermis is markedly thinned, the dermo-epidermal junction is largely effaced and there is more marked upper dermal fibrosis. Hypertrophic lesions show epidermal thickening similar to that seen in lichen simplex chronicus. The band-like infiltrate of LP is usually present, but the changes in hypertrophic LP can be less than entirely characteristic. In follicular LP, the infiltrate is grouped around the base of hair follicles with liquefaction degeneration in the external root sheath. There is often a plug in the mouth of the follicle.

Similar changes to those seen in the skin are also seen in oral LP, but it is important to note that a lichenoid histology is not uncommon in oral inflammation of whatever cause[19] and care should therefore be taken in interpreting oral biopsies. Shklar and McCarthy[19] believe that both clinical and pathological data must be taken together in making a diagnosis of oral LP.

What do all these changes represent? As already mentioned, basal cell degeneration seems to occur very early in LP. Electron microscopy has shown that there is disruption of the basement membrane with breaks and reduplication, with several attempts at new formation being made[22]. Experimental studies using $^{3}$H-labelled thymidine[24] suggest that the damaged basal cells are continuously replaced by cells migrating in from the edge of the LP lesion. However, the deliberate induction of a wound in LP papules[25] shows that cell replacement can also come from within the LP lesion itself. This has been supported by the work of Ebner and colleagues[26]. Although there have also been apparently paradoxical observations of reduced respiratory enzyme activity in the epidermis of LP papules[27], these findings imply that there is a continuous state of breakdown and repair of the basal layer occurring in LP.

What causes the basal cell damage? An infectious aetiology has been proposed for many years, but there is no real evidence that bacteria or viruses are directly responsible for the epidermal damage. However, immunopathological studies have suggested a mechanism by which these changes could occur.

## Immunopathology of lichen planus

The development of immunofluorescent techniques resulted in the discovery that immunoreactants were present in the lesions of LP[28]. The most constant findings are of fibrin in the upper dermis, along the basement membrane zone and around upper dermal vessels, and bright staining of what appear to be the cytoid bodies with immunoglobulins, especially IgM. Interestingly, this staining of cytoid body-like deposits is also seen in some biopsies from uninvolved skin[29]. However, it has also been stressed that these changes are by no means pathognomonic of LP and similar findings may be seen in biopsies from lupus erythematosus, eczema and other inflammatory dermatoses[29]. More recently, Olsen and colleagues[30] have reported the finding of an antigen specific to LP in the granular and prickle cell layers of the epidermis, using indirect immunofluorescence. The significance of this has yet to be established.

Monoclonal antobody studies have also been performed on the lesions of LP and it is now well established that the majority of the cells in the band-like infiltrate are T lymphocytes[31,32]. Further work has attempted to subdivide the infiltrating cells still further. It is clear that there are both T helper and T suppressor/cytotoxic subsets present in the infiltrate, although there has been some disagreement about the ratios[33]. The findings in at least three studies[33–35], however, are that there is a 2:1 ratio of helper to suppressor/cytotoxic subset in the dermal infiltrate, and that the cells seen infiltrating the epidermis are predominantly suppressor/cytotoxic T cells. It is also clear from this work that there are a large number of Langerhans cells present in both the dermis and epidermis in lesions of LP[33–35] and that epidermal keratinocytes express HLA-DR[36].

Some authors have claimed that there is also a systemic immunological disturbance in LP. For example, abnormal immunoglobulin levels have been reported on several occasions. However, two carefully controlled prospective studies have failed to confirm this[2,37], both failing to show any statistically significant variation in immunoglobulins from levels seen in normal controls. It has also been demonstrated that there is no increased incidence of autoimmune disease in patients with LP or in their relatives[2]. Mauduit and colleagues[38], however, have shown alterations in circulating T cell populations in patients with LP when examined before treatment commenced and again after one month[38]. These changes had disappeared by the end of the second month, suggesting that the changes were related to disease activity. There may also be depressed cell-mediated immune responses in LP[39].

The foregoing observations have led to increasing speculation that the lesions of LP are produced by immunopathological mechanisms and that the chain of events may begin with an assault on the basal cells by T-cells that are responding to altered epidermal antigenicity. Such alterations, it has been argued, may result from a variety of environmental triggers, including viral infections, drugs and chemicals. Such speculation has been fuelled further by the occurrence of LP and LP-like lesions in graft-versus-host reactions, as a reaction to some drugs, and in association with certain disorders that are thought to be autoimmune in origin. LP has also been associated with abnormal glucose tolerance.

## GRAFT-VERSUS-HOST DISEASE, LICHEN PLANUS-LIKE DRUG REACTIONS AND AUTOIMMUNE ASSOCIATIONS

### Graft-versus-host disease

This topic has been the subject of a recent review in this Series[40], and I shall therefore not dwell on it. However, the appearance of LP-like changes in early chronic graft-versus-host disease (GVHD) immediately generated much interest in graft-versus-host reactions as a model for idiopathic LP. The infiltrate in GVHD is generally sparser than that seen in LP and there are also differences in the pattern of the changes in the epidermis, but the fundamental feature of basal cell liquefaction is present. The cells infiltrating the epidermis are mostly T cells of the suppressor/cytotoxic subset, increasing speculation that they are responsible for the basal cell damage in both GVHD and LP. One interesting difference in the immunopathology of GVHD and LP is that Langerhans cells appear reduced in GVHD whereas, as we have seen, they are increased in number in early LP lesions[22].

## Lichen planus-like drug reactions

It became apparent during World War II that drugs are capable of inducing LP when many LP-like eruptions developed in servicemen taking mepacrine[41]. There are many other drugs that have been responsible, and a list of some of the more important offenders is given in Table 3.3. The lesions of drug-induced LP-like reactions may be clinically and histologically indistinguishable from idiopathic LP. In some instances, such as with the thiazides, the reactions may be light-induced, similar to the situation in LP actinicus. Gold may be responsible for a very severe and widespread reaction that can continue after the drug has been stopped. It is not known how these agents initiate the reaction, but it has been suggested that they may induce antigenic change in the skin or mucosae[42].

One very interesting drug is penicillamine. This agent is known to induce many different cutaneous reactions, including LP[43,44]. However, LP due to penicillamine is generally rare except in patients who are given the drug for primary biliary cirrhosis[45]. I shall return to this later.

TABLE 3.3 Important drugs and chemicals associated with LP-like reactions

| |
|---|
| Antimalarials |
| Quinine |
| Quinidine |
| $\beta$-Blockers |
| Phenothiazines |
| Gold |
| Chlorpropamide |
| $\alpha$-methyldopa |
| Thiazides (may be light-induced) |
| Penicillamine (particularly in patients with primary biliary cirrhosis) |
| Non-steroidal anti-inflammatory drugs (oral LP) |
| *P*-Phenylenediamine-derived colour developers (contact reaction) |

## Autoimmune disorders

There have been a number of reports associating LP with diseases in which autoimmunity is thought to play an important pathogenetic role, such as myasthenia gravis with thymoma, alopecia areata, vitiligo, ulcerative colitis and autoimmune liver disease[46]. There have also been reports of the association of LP with bullous pemphigoid[47] and, although some debate continues[14], it seems likely that this is a real phenomenon to be distinguished from bullous LP or LP pemphigoides.

Of particular interest is the relationship between LP and autoimmune liver disease. The first suggestion of a link between the two was made by Rebora and colleagues[48], who described five patients with erosive LP and liver disease. Subsequently, a series of patients from the Mayo Clinic was reported in whom penicillamine appeared to induce LP in patients with primary biliary cirrhosis[45]. However, a report from the Royal Free Hospital in London suggested that LP also occurred in patients with primary biliary cirrhosis independently of the administration of penicillamine[49]. Further analysis of the Mayo Clinic cases showed that this was indeed the case, although a majority of their cases of LP did appear to follow penicillamine therapy[50]. These patients, however, do seem to be a distinct subset, as two prospective studies have failed to show any evidence of liver disease in otherwise uncomplicated new cases of LP, both of skin and of mouth[2,51].

The interest generated by this observation of LP in patients with autoimmune liver disease, and particularly primary biliary cirrhosis, is heightened by the fact that Epstein and colleagues have pointed out several striking similarities between primary biliary cirrhosis and chronic graft-versus-host disease[52]. As has already been mentioned, LP lesions are common in patients with early chronic graft-versus-host disease. Indeed, Saurat[53] maintains that LP is the skin disease most closely mimicked by GVHD. Interestingly, Saurat also considers that some of the later changes of GVHD resemble lichen sclerosus et atrophicus, and we have[54] seen a patient with primary biliary cirrhosis and lichen sclerosus who also developed LP after penicillamine. These observations strongly suggest that the changes seen in LP, primary biliary cirrhosis and chronic graft-versus-host disease share common pathogenetic mechanisms[49].

### Abnormal glucose tolerance

One curious association that has been reported is the occurrence of abnormal glucose tolerance in 28 out of 33 patients with LP in one series[55], in 13 of 21 in another[56] and in 22 out of 40 in a third[57]. Jolly[55] considered that most of these patients had mild maturity-onset diabetes and Lowe and colleagues found that 42% of their patients had unequivocally abnormal glucose tolerance[57]. In Powell and colleagues' study[56] the changes were mild and consisted largely of high peak levels of blood glucose. Only four of their patients satisfied diagnostic criteria of diabetes mellitus. It remains unclear what the exact relationship is between LP and glucose intolerance, but it is certainly of some interest.

## TREATMENT OF LP

There are several indications for therapeutic intervention in LP. The skin lesions may be unsightly, but irritation is the commonest reason for a patient seeking advice about cutaneous LP. It is usually possible to control this with topical steroids, although agents in the potent (or group II) category are required. The addition of polythene occlusion may be of some help, especially in dealing with LP of the hands or feet. Hypertrophic LP may resist even the most potent of all topical steroids. Intralesional injections of triamcinolone are useful in this situation, as are ichthopaste bandages. Atrophic LP is difficult to treat. Topical steroids will suppress the inflammatory component but can also delay healing of ulcerated areas.

Occasionally, the irritation of cutaneous LP is so intense, and the eruption so widespread, that systemic therapy is required. The only drugs with a reliable and proven record are systemic steroids. I use oral prednisolone in moderately high dosage (40 mg a day) for a period of 2–3 weeks, reducing the dose thereafter and tailing off over about 2 months, depending on the response.

Oral lesions of LP are frequently asymptomatic. However, the mouth may be very sore and cause difficulty in eating. Topical steroid applications, as lozenges, oral pastes or sprays, may help, but bad oral LP often requires systemic steroids to bring it under control. Even after a course of systemic steroids, however, there are some patients who develop chronic changes in the mouth, usually of the atrophic type, that do not respond to anything. There are reports of responses of oral LP to griseofulvin and the retinoids, and these may be worth trying.

Nail changes are usually mild, but severe nail dystrophies in LP can lead to permanent loss and are another indication for systemic steroid therapy. Similarly, LP of the scalp may produce a widespread and permanent cicatricial alopecia: systemic steroids are essential if this is to be prevented.

## REFERENCES


1. Altman, J. and Perry, H. O. (1961). The variations and course of lichen planus. *Arch. Dermatol.*, **84,** 47–59
2. Shuttleworth, D., Graham-Brown, R. A. C. and Campbell, A. C. (1986). The autoimmune background in lichen planus. *Br. J. Dermatol.*, **115,** 199–203
3. Samman, P. D. (1961). Lichen planus. An analysis of 200 cases. *Trans. St John's Hosp. Dermatol. Soc.*, **46,** 36–38
4. Samman, P. D. (1979). Lichen planus. In Rook, A. Wilkinson, D. S. and Ebling, F. J. G. (eds.) *Textbook of Dermatology* 3rd Edn., pp. 1483–1496. (Oxford: Blackwell Scientific Publications)
5. Wilson, E. (1869). Leichen planus. *J. Cutan. Med.*, **3,** 117–132
6. Willan, R. (1808). *On Cutaneous Disease*, pp. 32–66. (London: J. Johnson).
7. Pinkus, H. (1973). Lichenoid tissue reactions. *Arch Dermatol.*, **107,** 840–846
8. Hebra, F. (1868). *On Diseases of the Skin, including the Exanthemata*, Vol II (translated and edited by C. Hilton Fagge and P. H. Pye-Smith). Reviewed in *J. Cutan. Med.*, **3,** 49–57 (1869)
9. Verhagen, A. R. H. B. and Koten, J. W. (1979). Lichenoid melanodermatitis. *Br. J. Dermatol.*, **101,** 651–658
10. Katzenellenbogen, I. (1962). Lichen planus actinicus (lichen planus in tropical countries). *Dermatologica*, **124,** 10–20
11. van der Schroeff, J. G., Schothorst, A. A. and Kanaar, P. (1983). Induction of actinic lichen planus with artificial UV sources. *Arch. Dermatol.*, **119,** 498–500
12. Sarkany, I., Caron, G. A. and Jones, H. A. (1964). Lichen planus pemphigoides. *Trans. St John's Hosp. Dermatol. Soc.*, **50,** 50–55
13. Sobel, S., Miller, R. and Shatin, H. (1976). Lichen planus pemphigoides. Immunofluorescent findings. *Arch. Dermatol.*, **112,** 1280–1283
14. Lang, P. G. and Maize, J. C. (1983). Co-existing lichen planus and bullous pemphigold or lichen planus pemphigoides? *J. Am. Acad. Dermatol.*, **9,** 133–140
15. Oomen, C., Temmerman, L. and Kint, A. (1986). Lichen planus pemphigoides. *Clin. Exp. Dermatol.*, **11,** 92–96
16. Kronenberg, K., Fretzin, D. and Potter, B. (1971). Malignant degeneration of lichen planus. *Arch. Dermatol.*, **104,** 304–307
17. Copeman, P. W. M., Schroeter, A. L. and Kierland, R. R. (1970). An unusual

variant of lupus erythematosus or lichen planus. *Br. J. Dermatol.*, **83,** 269–272
18. Davies, M. G., Gorkiewicz, A., Knight, A. and Marks, R. (1977). Is there a relationship between lupus erythematosus and lichen planus? *Br. J. Dermatol.*, **96,** 145–154
19. Shklar, G. and McCarthy (1961). The oral lesions of lichen planus. *Oral Surg., Oral Med., Oral Pathol.*, **14,** 164–181
20. Odukoya, O., Gallagher, G. and Shklar, G. (1985). A histologic study of epithelial dysplasia in oral lichen planus. *Arch. Dermatol.*, **121,** 1132–1136
21. Thyresson, N. and Moberger, G. (1957). Cytologic studies in lichen ruber planus. *Acta Dermatovenereol.*, **37,** 191–204
22. Sarkany, I. and Gaylarde, P. M. (1971). Ultrastructural and light microscopic changes of the epidermo-dermal junction. *Trans. St John's Hosp. Dermatol. Soc.*, **57,** 139–142
23. Ragaz, A. and Ackerman, A. B. (1981). Evolution, maturation and regression of lesions of lichen planus. *Am. J. Dermatopathol.*, **3,** 5–25
24. Marks, R., Black, M. and Wilson Jones, E. (1973). Epidermal cell kinetics in lichen planus. *Br. J. Dermatol.*, **88,** 37–45
25. Eady, R. A. J. and Cowan, T. (1977). Epidermal repair in lichen planus: a light and electron microscopical study. *Clin Exp. Dermatol.*, **2,** 323–334
26. Ebner, H., Gebhart, W., Lassmann, H. and Jurecka, W. (1976). The epidermal cell proliferation in lichen planus. *Acta Dermatovenereol.*, **56,** 1–4
27. Black, M. M. and Wilson Jones, E. (1972). The role of the epidermis in the histopathogenesis of lichen planus: Histochemical correlations. *Arch. Dermatol.*, **105,** 81–86
28. Baart de la Faille-Kuyer, E. H. and Baart de la Faille, H. (1974). An immunofluorescence study of lichen planus. *Br. J. Dermatol.*, **90,** 365–371
29. Abell, E., Presbury, D. G. C., Marks, R. and Ramnairam, D. (1975). The diagnostic significance of immunoglobulin and fibrin deposition in lichen planus. *Br. J. Dermatol.*, **93,** 17–24
30. Olsen, R. G., Du Plessis, D. P., Schulz, J. E. and Camisa, C. (1984). Indirect immunofluorescence microscopy of lichen planus. *Br. J. Dermatol.*, **110,** 9–15
31. Tan, R. S. H., Byrom, N. A. and Hayes, J. P. (1975). A method of liberating living cells from dermal infiltrate. Studies in skin reticuloses and lichen planus. *Br. J. Dermatol.*, **93,** 271–276
32. Bjerke, J. R. and Krogh, H. K. (1978). Identification of mononuclear cells *in situ* in skin lesions of lichen planus. *Br. J. Dermatol.*, **98,** 605–610
33. Matthews, J. B., Scully, C. M. and Potts, A. J. C. (1984). Oral lichen planus: an immunoperoxidase study using monoclonal antibodies to lymphocyte subsets. *Br. J. Dermatol.*, **111,** 587–595
34. Bhan, A. K., Harrist, T. J., Murphy, G. F. and Mihm, M. C. (1981). T cell subsets and Langerhans cells in lichen planus: *in situ* characterisation using monoclonal antibodies. *Br. J. Dermatol.*, **105,** 617–622
35. Bjerke, J. R. (1982). Subpopulations of mononuclear cells in lesions of psoriasis, lichen planus and discoid lupus erythematosus studied using monoclonal antibodies. *Acta Dermatovenereol.*, **62,** 477–483
36. Auböck, J., Romani, N., Grubauer, G. and Fritsch, P. (1986). HLA-DR expression on keratinocytes is a common feature of diseased skin. *Br. J. Dermatol.*, **114,** 465–472
37. Scully, C. (1982). Serum IgC, IgA, IgM, IgD and IgE in lichen planus: no evidence

for a humoral immunodeficiency. *Clin. Exp. Dermatol.*, **7,** 163–167
38. Mauduit, G., Fernandez-Bussy, R. and Thivolet, J. (1984). Sequential enumeration of peripheral blood T cell subsets in lichen planus. *Clin. Exp. Dermatol.*, **9,** 256–262
39. Shalid, J. and Marks, R. (1987). Depressed T cell mediated immunity in patients with lichen planus. *Br. J. Dermatol.*, **116,** 445–446
40. Harper, J. I. (1987). Graft vs host disease. In Verbov, J. L. (ed.) *Talking Points in Dermatology – I,* pp. 67–86. (Lancaster: MTP).
41. Feder, A. (1949). Clinical observations on atypical lichen planus and related dermatoses presumably due to atabrine toxicity. *Ann. Intern. Med.*, **31,** 1078–1089
42. Black, M. M. (1977). What is going on in lichen planus? *Clin. Exp. Dermatol.*, **2,** 303–310
43. Van de Staak, W. I. B. M., Cotton, D. W. K., Jonckheer-Venneste, M. M. H. and Boerbooms, A. M. T. H. (1975). Lichenoid eruption following penicillamine. *Dermatologica*, **150,** 372–374
44. Van Hecke, E., Kint, A. and Temmerman, L. (1981). A lichenoid eruption induced by penicilamine. *Arch. Dermatol.*, **117,** 676–677
45. Seehafer, J. R., Rogers, R. S., Fleming, C. R. and Dickson, E. R. (1981). Lichen planus-like lesions caused by penicillamine in primary biliary cirrhosis. *Arch. Dermatol.*, **117,** 140–142
46. Graham-Brown, R. A. C. (1986). Lichen planus and lichen planus-like reactions. *Br. J. Hosp. Med.*, **36,** 281–284
47. Stingl, G. and Holubar, K. (1975). Co-existence of lichen planus and bullous pemphigoid. *Br. J. Dermatol.*, **93,** 313–320
48. Rebora, A., Patri, R., Rampini, E., Crovato, F. and Ciravegna, G. (1978). Erosive lichen planus and cirrhotic hepatitis. *Ital. Gen. Rev. Dermatol.*, **2,** 123–127
49. Graham-Brown, R. A. C., Sarkany, I. and Sherlock, S. (1982). Lichen planus and primary biliary cirrhosis. *Br. J. Dermatol.*, **106,** 699–703
50. Powell, F. C., Rogers, R. S. and Dicksen, E. R. (1982). Lichen planus, primary biliary cirrhosis and penicillamine. *Br. J. Dermatol.*, **107,** 167
51. Möbacken, H., Nillson, L.-A., Olsson, R. and Sloberg, K. (1984). Incidence of liver disease in chronic lichen planus of the mouth. *Acta Dermatovenereol.*, **64,** 70–72
52. Epstein, O., Thomas, H. C. and Sherlock, S. (1980). Primary biliary cirrhosis is a dry gland syndrome with features of chronic graft-versus-host disease. *Lancet*, **1,** 1166–1168
53. Saurat, J. H. (1981). Cutaneous manifestations of graft-versus-host disease. *Int. J. Dermatol.*, **20,** 249–256
54. Graham-Brown, R. A. C. and Sarkany, I. (1986). Lichen sclerosus et atrophicus with primary biliary cirrhosis and lichen planus. *Int. J. Dermatol.*, **25,** 317
55. Jolly, M. (1972). Lichen planus and its association with diabetes mellitus. *Med. J. Austr.*, **1,** 990–992
56. Powell, S. M., Ellis, J. P., Ryan, T. J. and Vickers, H. R. (1974). Glucose tolerance in lichen planus. *Br. J. Dermatol.*, **91,** 73–75
57. Lowe, N. J., Cudworth, A. G., Clough, S. A. and Bullen, M. F. (1976). Carbohydrate metabolism in lichen planus. *Br. J. Dermatol.*, **95,** 9–12

# 4

# JUVENILE PLANTAR DERMATOSIS

*R. M. GRAHAM*

## INTRODUCTION

Since the late 1960s, an uncomfortable and often sore condition affecting the weight-bearing surface of children's feet has become recognized as a distinct clinical entity. It is characterized by shiny, cracked and peeling skin, involving predominantly the plantar surface of the forefoot. It is the commonest form of dermatitis to affect the soles of children's feet in the UK.

There have been accounts of juvenile plantar dermatosis (JPD) occurring prior to the 1960s and, although these reports are largely anecdotal, comments from some of our patients' parents offer some support to this. However, it is only fair to say that if it occurred before the 1960s, it was by comparison a very uncommon condition! The more frequent occurrence appears to be at least temporally associated with changes from traditional leather footwear to synthetic, purportedly more modern, occlusive counterparts. The first description in the literature was in 1968 by Silvers and Glickman[1]. In 1972, both Enta[2] in Canada and Möller[3] in Sweden described separate series of almost similar cases, and together with Silvers and Glickman[1] they considered it to be an irritant-type contact eczema related to footwear, friction and sweating; a condition to which the atopic child appeared particularly prone. While Möller's paper[3] was still in press, Schultz and Zachariae[4], published the results of tests suggesting that atopy was not implicated in the disorder, which they termed 'recurrent juvenile eczema of the hands and feet'. The importance of the various possible aetiological factors in JPD has remained controversial, as has the underlying pathophysiology of the condition.

## TERMINOLOGY

The term juvenile plantar dermatosis (JPD) was first used by MacKie and Hussain in 1976[5] and is now the generally accepted term for the condition. Other names that have been used are 'forefoot eczema'[6], 'atopic winter feet'[3], 'peridigital dermatitis'[2], 'dermatitis plantaris sicca'[7], 'la pulpite seche de l'avant-pied'[8] and 'wet and dry foot syndrome'[9]. The 'sweaty sock dermatitis' described by Gibson in 1963[10] bears some resemblance to JPD, but the description of interdigital involvement and vesiculation, suggest that a different dermatosis is described.

## APPEARANCE

The skin on the plantar surface of the foot becomes shiny, losing its normal dermatoglyphics, and takes on a 'collodion' or 'cellophane-like' appearance. This almost 'plastic-like' smooth surface becomes fissured to a variable extent, with splits of dry scaly skin, giving a crazy-paving finish (Figure 4.1). These fissures, particularly when occurring on the lateral margins of the feet, become deep and prone to bleeding. The cracks, when severe, are sore to walk on and may necessitate time off school and sporting activities. Sometimes, shallow fissures become ingrained with dirt and give a black 'criss-crossed' appearance to the sole (Figure 4.2), but more commonly they remain powdery white and give rise to foci of peeling skin. If these are traumatized, they can cause considerable discomfort and commonly bleed.

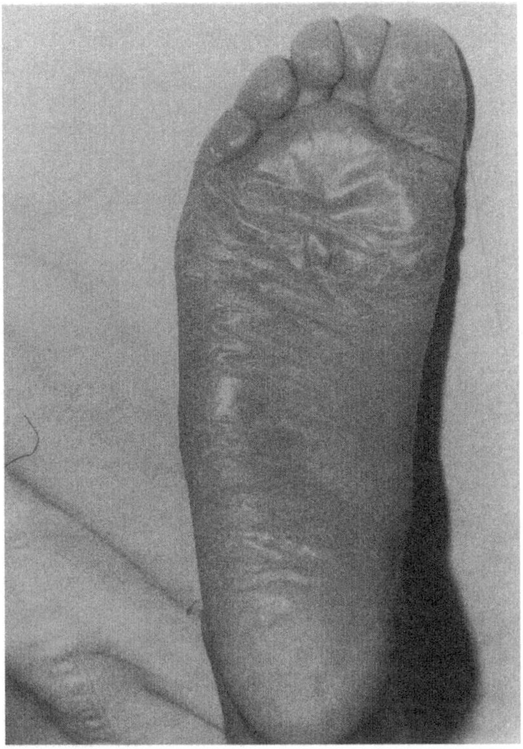

FIGURE 4.1 Cracking of skin with a background shiny, collodion-like appearance in JPD. Note sparing of arch

## DISTRIBUTION

The eruption is normally symmetrical in distribution, but occasionally one foot may be much more severely affected, such that it can appear unilateral. When this occurs, the dominant side generally shows the greater involvement; presumably owing to greater frictional forces affecting that foot.

In about 60% of cases, involvement is limited to the plantar surface of the forefoot (Figure 4.3), but additional heel involvement is seen in approximately 40%[11] (Figure 4.4). The distribution is usually within the pattern that a bare footprint makes on the floor, i.e. omitting the arch of the foot and the flexor surface of the shafts of the toes; this

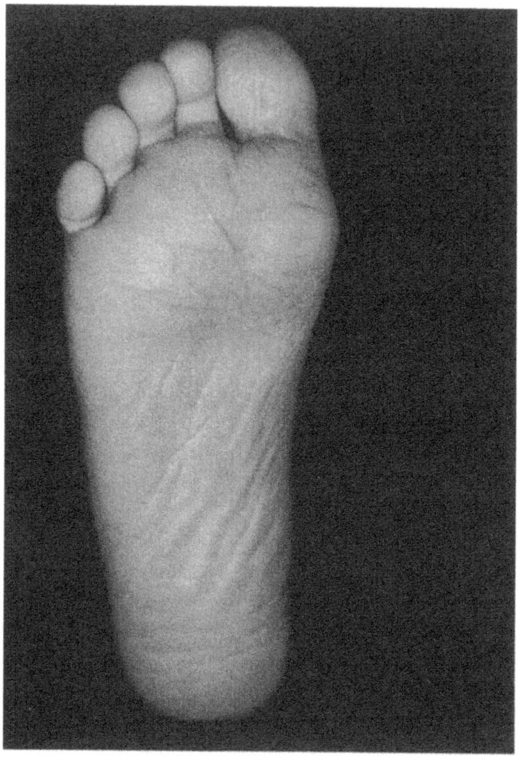

FIGURE 4.2 Black criss-crossed appearance in JPD. Note the sparing of the heel and the pads of all the toes except the big toe

corresponds with the sites of maximum friction and humidity on the foot. The interdigital spaces are usually unaffected. However, the distribution may vary, from exacerbation to exacerbation, within the same individual. Occasionally the changes extend onto the dorsum of the toes and this is generally accepted as an indication to exclude allergic contact eczema[12].

We have found[11], as have other workers[2,4,13,14], that a small group of patients also show similar changes on their fingertips and hands (Figures 4.5 and 4.6). All of the cases we have seen with this distribution have had heel involvement and have also been atopic; the numbers, however, have been small (eight) and this association could have occurred by chance. Isolated heel involvement is not normally

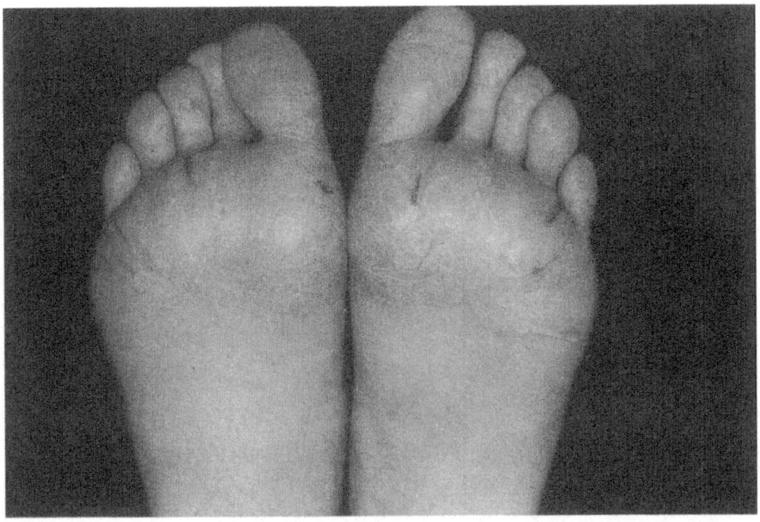

FIGURE 4.3 Typical forefoot involvement in JPD, with deep fissures that bleed

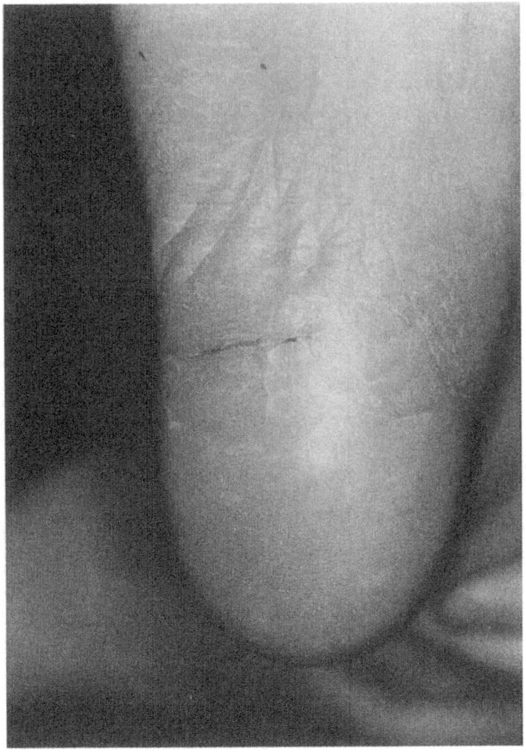

FIGURE 4.4 Anterior heel involvement in JPD

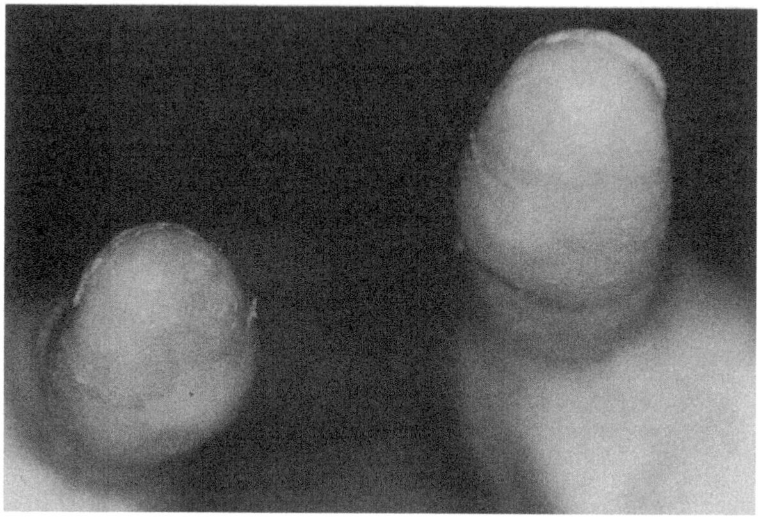

FIGURE 4.5 Thumb involvement in JPD. Note similar peeling of skin

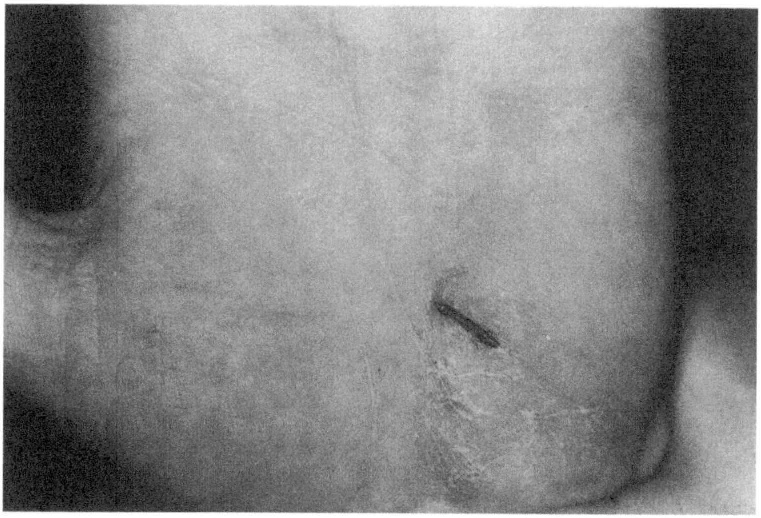

FIGURE 4.6 Palm involvement in JPD. Note similar cracking and fissuring

seen, but I have seen a child in whom forefoot involvement had virtually resolved, but whose heels remained affected. The clinical appearances of fingertip, thenar and hypothenar eminence involvement is similar to that of JPD, with dryness, fissuring and peeling of the skin, but is indistinguishable from an irritant hand eczema, or dermatitis palmaris sicca described by Lim *et al.* in 1986[15]. It is impossible, therefore, to distinguish these changes from an irritant hand eczema in an atopic patient.

## AGE RANGE

The condition usually starts at 5–6 years of age, often coinciding with the commencement of infant schooling; there is, however, considerable variation in the starting age. Cases have been documented of its appearance soon after birth, before the wearing of footwear and before the onset of walking[16]. The problem has rarely been described in adults; an Australian report[17] describes a 30-year-old Vietnamese refugee unaccustomed to wearing shoes, who developed JPD after commencing to wear 'Western-type' footwear when relocated in Australia. The oldest patient that I have seen with JPD was aged 19 years; it normally clears between 11 and 15 years of age irrespective of treatment. Whether this is related to, or just coincidentally linked with, puberty is uncertain. It may resolve much earlier than puberty, but such cases are prone to relapse, presumably if the feet are subjected to the aggravating environmental factors.

## SEX DISTRIBUTION AND INCIDENCE

Accurate figures on the incidence of JPD are not available. Friis[7] in 1973 felt that it was the commonest dermatitis to affect the feet of children in Denmark; certainly this is still the case in Merseyside. However, several of our dermatological colleagues have commented that fewer cases are now being referred compared with the early 1980s. Whilst this may represent an actual change in incidence, feasibly related to improvements in footwear, an alternative explanation is that many cases are now diagnosed and managed in general practice.

Virtually all of the reports involving substantial numbers of children with JPD have shown that there is a slight male preponderance[11,18,19]. In general, the condition appears to start earlier, and to persist longer, in boys than girls[11]. The easy explanation for this is that boys' feet are subjected to more frictional trauma in activities such as football, etc., and perhaps that they are more likely to wear occlusive synthetic footwear, than girls. This, however, is pure speculation and no direct evidence exists that this is the case. However, Stankler[20] felt that the only difference between identical twin girls, one of whom had marked involvement with JPD and the other minimal affliction, was that the former was a 'tomboy'.

Moorthy and Rajan[21], commented on a more persistent group, who are mainly female and non-atopic, in whom the disorder starts at puberty and persists into the late teens. It might at first seem that this may be related to the wearing of tight fitting, occlusive, high-heeled footwear, but their study does not confirm this.

## SEASONAL OCCURRENCE

Silvers and Glickman[1] felt that JPD was exacerbated by perspiration experienced in hot weather, but Möller[3] felt that cold weather was implicated, so much so that it was called 'atopic winter feet'. Some workers have felt that it was related to extreme perspiration and friction in winter footwear, followed by rapid drying, when removing footwear in a household of low humidity[2]. MacKie and Hussain[5], by comparison, found no distinct seasonal pattern and this is my overall finding. However, within this generalization, in the cases I have studied, approximately 25% underwent primarily winter exacerbations and a similar percentage flared in the summer, with 50% fluctuating irrespective of season[11]. Although this difference in seasonal findings may appear conflicting, Steck[9] found, in California, that JPD was worse in the summer and he suggested that the worldwide difference in seasonal variation is due to a rapid alteration between the extremes of wet and dry affecting the stratum corneum.

## SWEATING

Although it is evident that in established JPD there is a reduction in active sweat glands in the affected areas, demonstrated using a 5% *o*-phthaldialdehyde in xylene sweat test, there does seem to be a group of patients who claim to have suffered from hyperhidrosis prior to the onset of JPD. This is not usually visible on the affected plantar surface of the foot when the dermatosis is active, but may be observed on the unaffected hands or arch of the foot. I have found this to be a complaint in up to a third of cases, with about 10% having visible hyperhidrosis. Ashton and Griffiths[22], in a study on sweating, have confirmed that there is a reduction in active sweat duct openings on the affected areas of big toes, but they were unable to demonstrate an increase or decrease in sweat retention compared to controls. Unfortunately the interpretation of this latter finding must be circumspect, as assessing for hyperhidrosis in a condition that is known to develop hypohidrosis as it develops is fraught with problems, and may be impossible. Molokhia[23] has interpreted his findings of only slight difference between sweat production between JPD sufferers and controls' feet as an indication of likely localized hyperhidrosis in the condition, as more than half of the sole in JPD is by comparison anhidrotic.

## DIAGNOSIS

This is generally made on the clinical appearance, location and circumstances of the individual case, as described previously. The condition tends to be sore or painful, rather than itchy, although I have found that up to 20% of cases do complain of itching. The relative uncommonness of itch as a symptom has been suggested as clinical evidence that JPD is a non-eczematous disorder[19], but whilst one would agree that vesiculation, a feature of acute eczema, is never seen, itch, a common symptom of eczema, tends to be a sensation overridden by pain or discomfort. This is further supported by the fact that other analogous processes such as 'housewife's' irritant hand eczema are seldom vesicular and not always itchy, but often sore.

Rarely JPD can present with acute inflammation, swelling and discharge; the child usually finds weight-bearing painful and is reluctant to allow examination of the feet. This virtually always represents an infective exacerbation, in which bacteria, usually streptococci, have gained access to the tissues via the fissuring to produce a cellulitis of the foot. When this presents, it is not always easy to discern the underlying JPD, as this is camouflaged by erythema, oedema and crusting.

## PERSONAL HISTORY ATOPY (TABLE 4.1)

The incidence of atopy has varied from 94% in Silvers and Glickman's original report[1] to 0% in Shrank's series[24]. This may be explained in part by the imprecise definition of atopy. We have taken this to be delineated by a personal history of asthma, atopic eczema or hay fever and similar histories in first-degree relatives. Whilst one of our colleagues originally described the condition as atopic eczema localized to the forefoot[25], we all agree that whilst the majority of our cases are atopic (58%), there is a group who do not have a known association with this state.

TABLE 4.1 Comparative incidence of atopy in previous series

| Study | Atopic history (%) | | | Number in series |
|---|---|---|---|---|
| | Personal | Family | Combined | |
| Silvers & Glickman, 1968 [1] | 27 | 67 | 94 | 15 |
| Enta, 1972 [2] | 29 | — | 61 | 52 |
| Möller, 1972 [3] | 31 | 54 | 92 | 13 |
| Mackie and Hussain, 1976 [5] | 12 | 11 | 22 | 102 |
| Shrank, 1978 [24] | 0 | 0 | 0 | 38 |
| Moorthy and Rajan, 1984 [21] | 8 | 22 | 42 | 64 |
| Young, 1986 [19] | 25 | 32 | 43 | 28 |
| Ashton and Griffiths, 1986 [36] | 30 | 43 | 61 | 250 |
| Jones *et al.*, 1987 [33] | 30 | 42 | 42 | 50 |
| Graham *et al.*, 1987 [11] | 48 | 52 | 58 | 98 |

* Reference numbers in brackets

This controversy is further compounded by the finding that, in the cases that have had atopic eczema, this has seldom been or seldom is severe. Also, the atopic state does not appear to give rise to a more severe form of JPD, compared with the non-atopic group, nor does it persist longer. It has been suggested that children with active atopic eczema are less active in terms of running, etc., and so are less likely to incur frictional forces that might precipitate JPD. An alternative theory would be that all cases share a predisposition to irritant contact eczema, but not all express atopic manifestations. It is my belief that this predisposition is inherited, but that environmental factors may modify its expression. This is further supported by the fact that not all the families with two siblings affected are atopic.

It is my experience that serum IgE estimations, RAST tests and prick tests have proved of only limited value in discerning those who have a background of atopy and those who have not. These tests tend to be positive in those with active atopy, but if a child has a past history of atopy that has subsequently resolved, the tests are frequently negative.

## FAMILY HISTORY OF JPD

In Merseyside we have found an approximately 25% incidence of a family history of JPD and, whilst most of the cases are with sibling involvement, we are now starting to see involvement in the next generation. Anecdotally, several parents have commented that grandparents of the child have claimed to have also suffered from the condition in their childhood. Like Stankler[20], we have also seen the condition in both of identical twins, as well as in both of non-identical twins.

## SPORT

There does not appear to be an obvious sporting association, although in a condition of irritant dermatitis in which frictional forces are one of the exacerbating factors, intensive exercise is likely to increase soreness, cracking and subsequent bleeding. One has to qualify these comments by adding that many children are naturally reluctant to implicate their favourite sporting pastimes as an aggravating factor in their dermatosis, in case they are subsequently prevented from pursuing the activity. Some authorities[9,24] have found that swimming may aggravate the condition and this would fit with Steck's[9] causal theory of rapid alteration between wet and dry states of the stratum corneum. I have found swimming to be implicated in only four of our cases.

## FOOTWEAR

Hole[26] has pointed out that the disposal of sweat from the foot is inhibited by footwear, and that leather is effective in absorbing and transmitting water vapour from the environment of the foot. The water vapour permeability varies from 7.4 mg/cm/h for calf leather to 1.1 mg/cm/h for Corfam, to less than 0.05 mg/cm/h for PVC woven cotton fabrics. The use of anti-scuff agents on the outside of footwear and of polymer shoe linings will also inhibit the transmission of water vapour through the shoe. This inability to dispose of humidity may result in pooling of liquid under or around the sole. If the socks are relatively non-absorbent and synthetic in nature, the liquid will remain contained around the foot in a similar fashion to a sponge. The result of this will be that the skin of the plantar surface will be saturated for long periods of time. It is of interest that the dampest part of the foot also coincides with the pressure points on the plantar surface, which are also the sites of greatest friction. Absorbent socks, such as cotton socks, act via a wicking effect to disperse liquid out of the shoe and it may be that long cotton socks may be more effective in this respect than short socks[27]. It is not surprising, therefore, that JPD has been linked with the introduction of predominantly synthetic footwear in the 1960s, a time when it became fashionable for 'trainers' to be worn, providing an environment in which effects of friction and humidity may be encountered.

Unfortunately, once the condition has developed, change of footwear to absorbent socks and shoes with leather uppers, does not necessarily resolve the condition, and in fact 75% of our patients felt that appropriate footwear changes had not significantly helped the disorder. Up to 24% of our parents claimed that their children were wearing appropriate footwear prior to the problem developing. One should bear several qualifications in mind when interpreting this data. (1) It is largely anecdotal information that one obtains when retrospectively enquiring about footwear worn when the eruption started. (2) Parents are naturally reluctant to accept that there is any deficiency in the footwear that they have provided for their child. (3) Information may be forthcoming about the 'best' shoes the child has, rather than trainers the child has for 'out of school hours' and playing.[4] Even when directly examining footwear, it is often difficult for 'professionals', let alone parents, to be certain of their suitability.

When advising parents on suitable footwear for their child it is worth discussing discreetly with the parent what sort of footwear the child is going to accept. This is particularly relevant when one considers that changes are likely to improve rather than cure the condition and that the purchase of often expensive footwear may represent a considerable financial burden on the family. We have seen several children who have flatly refused to wear anything but trainers for fear of ostracism from their peer group; probably for similar reasons, two of our patients have claimed that the problem is aggravated by wearing anything but trainers. In such circumstances, it is worth suggesting that parents investigate what is the least-occlusive and best-ventilated type, available in the style that the child will accept. Whilst leather soles may be the best material for the dispersal of plantar humidity, they are impractical for recommendation in children, on the grounds of being insufficiently durable, expensive and not readily obtainable. Although sandals are often helpful in the summer months, they are not always acceptable to the child and I have seen several patients with exacerbations of their JPD following the wearing of sandals. In fact, those familiar with wearing sandals will realize that it is possible to get free pooling of sweat on the insole of a sandal, particularly in hot weather; this demonstrates the limitation that ventilation of the uppers can have on plantar humidity!

In general, I recommend purchase of shoes with synthetic soles, permeable non-synthetic insoles (cork or leather) and soft leather uppers, preferably unfinished on the inner surface, avoiding impermeable linings and anti-scuff or highly glossed exterior surfaces. This usually means 'buckskin' or suede-like shoes. However, the limitations of the likely benefits should be explained to the parents before they embark on such purchases; it is of interest that on follow-up of our patients more have claimed benefit from the change of their synthetic nylon socks to either cotton or less frequently wool socks, than from changes in their shoes. Socks containing 85% cotton are generally adequate, more robust and readily available, compared with the pure cotton varieties. Shoes should also be allowed to dry out, before wearing again; so if possible, a change of suitable footwear is useful. Advice on footwear should be tempered by flexibility of schools footwear regulations, the ability of the parent to understand the information imparted and the affordability of such changes.

## HISTOLOGY AND PATHOPHYSIOLOGY

The information available on the histopathological changes in JPD are limited by the modest number of reports containing histological findings. When pathological studies have been performed, only small numbers of cases have been involved. This is likely to be due to the natural reluctance to perform biopsies on the soles of children's feet in a condition that is normally readily diagnosed clinically.

Shrank[24] examined serial sections from the ball of the foot of two patients demonstrating mild acanthosis with little parakeratosis or dermal infiltrate, but evidence of focal spongiosis around the sweat duct in the Malpighian layer. He noticed sweat duct changes, mainly in the horny layer, with ductal narrowing and blockage by PAS-positive material, together with lateral displacement of ducts. He inferred that this reflected a process allied to a chronic miliaria-like condition, that resulted when high-humidity conditions were encountered inside occlusive footwear; possibly aggravated by shearing forces acting on the foot of an energetic child. Van Dijk *et al.*[13] examined the histopathological changes from the lateral margin of one patient's foot, which showed hyperkeratosis, localized parakeratosis, acanthosis and some spongiosis. There was a slight dermal, mononuclear perivascular infiltrate and papillary oedema. He concluded that these changes were consistent with a picture of asteatotic eczema.

Kint *et al.*[28] reported histological findings on one case, revealing a hyperkeratotic but also orthokeratotic stratum corneum, a normal stratum granulosum and a slightly acanthotic spinous cell layer, with elongation of the rete ridges and a few spongiotic areas. They found a normal basal layer and deep dermis, but the capillaries in the papillary dermis were surrounded by a lymphocytic and histiocytic infiltrate. Maleville and coworkers[8] managed to examine three cases, finding in the epidermis orthokeratosis, areas of hypergranulosis and a tendency towards papillomatosis. In the dermis, there was a discrete non-specific infiltrate. In one of their samples, several foci of spongiosis were observed, with exocytosis of polymorphonuclear lymphocyte cells, but without microabscess formation or parakeratotic changes that would point towards psoriasis.

Ashton and colleagues[14] have performed the most extensive and detailed histopathological survey, involving six patients. In all cases, a sparse upper dermal mononuclear cell infiltrate was present, occasionally localized around the intradermal portion of the sweat duct, but mostly just below the sweat duct entry into epidermis. Hypogranulosis and parakeratosis were observed, together with irregular and psoriasiform acanthosis. Inflammatory changes within the epidermis were mainly acrosyringeal, most cases showing paranuclear vacuolization of keratinocytes, spongiosis and a sparse mononuclear cell infiltrate. They concluded that there was little evidence to suggest that the pathophysiology of JPD was miliaria-like, but the changes in JPD were consistent with an eczematous process.

Steck's[9] theory of the pathomechanics is that saturation and desaturation of the keratin layer produces minor cellular damage to the skin, which is negligible unless the drying occurs rapidly, when rupture of cellular bonds leads to a rent in the fabric of the superficial layers of skin and, as a consequence, to even more rapid drying.

A frequently quoted[14,18] study by Stewart[29] demonstrating sweat duct occlusion, sweat retention and spongiosis, was, in fact, describing histological changes in an irritant hand eczema affecting the right hand of women, rather than JPD. In the absence of further confirmatory reports of Shrank's[24] miliarial findings, the overall described changes are reasonably consistent with, and suggestive of, an eczematous process with a non-specific, often peri-sweat duct inflammatory infiltrate and secondary reactive changes in the stratum corneum. Shrank's[24] observations, however, should not be discounted, as the repertory of evidence is small and relative anhidrosis is an undoubted sequela of the process. Certainly, it has been demonstrated that miliaria and anhidrosis can be produced experimentally[30] after 48 hours occlusion of skin with 'Saran Wrap' (cling film). The histological changes are similar to some of those described in JPD by Shrank[24]. What does seem controversial is the interpretation of these findings: although oedema, maceration and shearing forces acting on the keratin and acrosyringium may produce sweat duct occlusion, it is argued that this is not the primary process[14]. This unfortunately results in a rather unproductive, 'cause and effect' argument that, in being unresolvable, is probably best avoided. Perhaps the analogy with Stewarts' irritant housewife's hand eczema[29] was a Freudian slip that has much to commend it!

Mackie[18] points out that there have been no particular technical problems with any of the children biopsied to date and it does not therefore seem unreasonable to consider biopsy in the more severe or intractable cases, so that histological findings can be confirmed; electron microscopy and immunotyping could also be performed. Understandably, ethical committees are reluctant to approve such studies, particularly in the children's hospital situation, which is the only environment in which sufficient, severe cases are likely to be encountered.

## MYCOLOGY AND BACTERIOLOGY

The commonest diagnostic mistake in JPD by the practitioner is that of a fungal infection of the feet; with the finding that the condition is unresponsive to antifungal agents, the case is then often referred. Treatment, under such circumstances, has nearly always been empirical, mycological specimens rarely having been examined. However, in prepubertal children, tinea pedis infections are exceptionally uncommon[12]. In fact, all mycology performed on our cases has proved negative; although it is possible for the older child to has co-existent tinea pedis, we have not yet seen this. These observations coincide with those of most other workers with experience of this condition[18,9]. Despite this uncommon incidence of fungal infections, interdigital scaling and maceration would be indications for mycological examination. Ashton and Griffiths[22] have examined for bacteria in JPD and have found no difference between control and JPD groups in terms of colonies cultured, and in bacterial counts, which are usually either of *Staphylococcus albus*, or *S. pyogenes*.

## ALLERGIC CONTACT SENSITIVITY

It is generally accepted that allergic contact dermatitis seldom occurs in young children (0–4 years), although the incidence appears to increase gradually with age, so that in the 10–15 age group it is not an uncommon event[31,32]. The distribution pattern of juvenile plantar dermatosis might suggest an aetiology of an allergic contact eczema. However, the majority of studies have demonstrated a low incidence of relevant positive patch-test results[33,11]. There have been exceptions to this: thus, White and coworkers[34] found 11 out of 13 children had significant patch-test findings, two of which were to synthetic constituents of their shoes. Hanifein[35], in 1978, described a specific shoe dermatitis, due to an allergic contact sensitivity to an adhesive used in a well-known make of training shoe. The distribution, age group and appearance of this eruption is not described, but the inference is that it was seen in (presumably?) adult joggers, rather than in children.

In a study of foot dermatitis performed by Weston *et al.*[12] it was demonstrated that distribution is the major clue to identifying those children with foot dermatoses related to allergic contact sensitivity. They found that if the dermatosis extended onto the dorsum of the foot, there was a 42% incidence of allergic contact eczema, whereas those with involvement of the weight-bearing surfaces alone (JPD) had a zero incidence. They also found that, with avoidance procedures, those children with an identifiable allergen could remain disease-free. This makes the occurrence of a dermatitis on the dorsum of a child's foot, a very strong indication for patch testing.

By contrast, Mackie[18] found a 10% incidence of positive patch tests to one or more constituents of footwear in their tested cases of JPD; retrospective analysis of these did not reveal any useful distinguishing features between JPD and allergic footwear dermatitis.

Obviously, the development of JPD soon after the purchase of a certain pair of shoes is another positive indication for patch testing, as may be other clinical features that suggest a deviation from the normal pattern of JPD.

Of the published reports, where reasonable numbers of patients have been patch-tested, results can be divided into those that are thought to be relevant to a dermatitis on the feet and those that are coincidental findings; mercaptobenzothiazole, mercapto-mix and chromate seem to be the commonest pertinent, positive results[12,36].

In Liverpool we have patch-tested approximately one fifth of the 140 cases we have now followed up, the majority of these cases have shown either some extension onto the dorsum of the foot or an exacerbation with certain footwear. A conventional patch-testing technique is employed using a standard European battery, a special shoe battery, together with samples from uppers, inners and soles of the patient's shoes. Only three positive findings have been obtained – parabens (1) nickel (2) – and none of these is likely to be related to footwear, although parabens may have been a preservative in a topical treatment administered for JPD. A list of possible allergens for a special shoe battery is given in Table 4.2, although in general it is our experience that in the majority of cases of JPD patch testing is unhelpful.

What is surprising is that more cases of allergic contact dermatitis of the feet are not seen. In JPD, the combination of often sweaty feet and cracked skin covered by materials containing dyes, preservatives, rubbers, glues and metals would seem the ideal environment for contact sensitization to occur.

## TREATMENT

The best approach to the management of JPD is to explain the nature of the problem, in easily understood terms, to the parents. Unless this is done, parents will return dissatisfied when all the appropriate changes in footwear and topical therapies have been made but the dermatosis persists. Once parents understand that the nature of the condition is variable, that it only completely resolves in the teens, and that recommendations only assist but do not cure the problem, then greater mutual understanding and cooperation can be achieved.

The majority of patients/parents that I have questioned with regard

TABLE 4.2 Comprehensive battery including dilutions and vehicles for patch testing foot dermatoses

| *Compound* | *Concentration* | *Vehicle* |
|---|---|---|
| Glutaraldehyde | 1% | Aqueous |
| Formaldehyde* | 1% | Aqueous |
| Potassium dichromate* | 0.5% | Petrolatum |
| Nickel sulphate* | 5% | Petrolatum |
| Cobalt chloride* | 1% | Petrolatum |
| Phenyl mercuric nitrate | 0.05% | Aqueous |
| Epoxy resin* | 1% | Petrolatum |
| Lanolin (wool alcohols)* | 30% | Petrolatum |
| Colophony* | 20% | Petrolatum |
| Parabens* | 15% | Petrolatum |
| Chlorocresol | 1% | Petrolatum |
| Resorcinol | 1% | Petrolatum |
| Kathon CG | 0.02% | Aqueous |
| Paraphenylenediamine* | 0.5% | Petrolatum |
| Ethylenediamine hydrochloride* | 1% | Petrolatum |
| Hydroquinone monobenzyl ether | 1% | Petrolatum |
| *Para*-tert-butylphenolformaldehyde resin | 1% | Petrolatum |
| *Para*-tert-butylphenol | 2% | Petrolatum |
| *Para*-aminoazobenzene | 0.25% | Petrolatum |
| Carbamix* | 3% | Petrolatum |
| 1,3-diphenylguanidine | 0.5% | Petrolatum |
| Zinc diethydithiocarbamate | 0.5% | Petrolatum |
| Zinc dibutyldithiocarbamate | 0.5% | Petrolatum |
| Black rubber mix* | 0.6% | Petrolatum |
| *N*-isopropyl-*N*-phenyl-4-phenylenediamine | 0.1% | Petrolatum |
| *N*-cyclohexyl-*N*-phenyl-4-phenylenediamine | 0.25% | Petrolatum |
| *N,N*-diphenyl-4-phenylenediamine | 0.25% | Petrolatum |
| Mercaptomix* | 2% | Petrolatum |
| *N*-cyclohexylbenzothiazyl sulphenamide | 0.5% | Petrolatum |
| Mercaptobenzothiazole | 0.5% | Petrolatum |
| Morpholinylmercaptobenzothiazole | 0.5% | Petrolatum |
| Thiuram mix* | 1% | Petrolatum |
| Tetramethylthiuram monosulphide | 0.25% | Petrolatum |
| Tetramethylthiuram disulphide | 0.25% | Petrolatum |
| Tetraethylthiuram disulphide | 0.25% | Petrolatum |
| Diphenylthiourea | 1% | Petrolatum |
| Diethylthiourea | 1% | Petrolatum |
| Ethylbutylthiourea (subject to availability) | 1% | Petrolatum |
| *N,N*-diphenylguanidine | 1% | Petrolatum |
| Dodecylmercaptan | 0.1% | Petrolatum |
| *N*-butylacrylate | 2% | Petrolatum |
| 2-n-octyl-4-isothiazolin-3-one | 0.1% | Petrolatum |
| Disperse orange 3 | 1% | Petrolatum |
| Acid yellow 36 | 1% | Petrolatum |
| Disperse brown 1 | 1% | Petrolatum |
| Vegetable tans (subject to availability) | 1% | Petrolatum |

* In European standard battery

to the efficacy of topical therapy have felt that preparations were generally ineffective. On further questioning, a common complaint was that, although treatments may help initially, benefit was not maintained despite continued usage[11].

A list of the commonly used and helpful preparations is given in Table 4.3. However, virtually any emollient will be of some help. Conventional topical steroids only appear as good as their emollient base; a common complaint is that they cause stinging, especially when potent and used in a cream formulation. For general use, white or yellow soft paraffin, with or without 5% salicylic acid is one of the more beneficial preparations, but suffers from the disadvantage of leaving the feet feeling sticky. The best preparation I have found, which was recommended to me by the late Dr Ian Sneddon, is a porous, heavy-duty, lubricating hand cream that is commercially available without prescription (Neutrogena Hand Cream)[37]. This seems as good as white soft paraffin and is cosmetically more acceptable. Steck[9] has

TABLE 4.3 Common treatments for JPD

| *Treatment* | *Comments* |
|---|---|
| Porous lubricating hand cream* | Available over the counter, pleasant to use, but contains fragrance and parabens |
| White soft paraffin (±5–10% salicylic acid†) | Leaves feet feeling 'tacky'; salicylic acid sometimes stings. |
| Preparations containing 10% urea† | Often causes stinging, but if tolerated often helpful |
| White's tar paste/tar paste bandages | Messy and smelly, but can be soothing and helpful |
| Topical steroids | Routinely only as good as emollient base, except perhaps in exacerbations, when the treatment below is probably the best application |
| Hydrocortisone-impregnated and zinc-paste bandages | Occlusion with both is helpful in exacerbations |

* Neutrogena Norwegian Formula Hand Cream, Neutrogena (UK) Ltd.
† Salicylic acid and urea preparations can promote rotting of footwear, especially of cotton.

pointed out that preparations should be applied immediately after removing footwear and after bathing; I would agree with this and would additionally recommend application prior to putting on footwear.

If JPD is about to undergo an exacerbation, then conventional topical therapies will appear ineffective or even to exacerbate the problem. If the feet become very sore, hydrocortisone (in Cortacream) and zinc oxide bandages (Viscopaste PB7) used in combination are very helpful. On the very rare occasions that cellulitis or other secondary bacterial infection develops, systemic antibiotics are indicated, infection may warrant hospital admission. It is of interest that children otherwise hospitalized and confined to bed usually undergo either an improvement or temporary resolution of their JPD[24].

## COURSE AND OUTCOME

The mean age of resolution of our cases is currently 12.3 years, with a mean duration of approximately 7 years. Males seem to suffer for marginally longer than females, but there does not appear to be a difference between the atopic and non-atopic groups. The majority of our cases have cleared by the age of 14 years; those that have cleared very early have tended to relapse again prior to adolescence; we have several cases that have lasted until 16 years of age and one up to 19 years. In these latter cases, even though the dermatosis persists, in general it causes little discomfort. One of the most pleasing features of JPD is to be able to reassure parents and patients that virtually all cases will resolve by or at some time during adolescence.

## Acknowledgements

I would like to thank Dr Clodagh King, Consultant Dermatologist in charge of the Patch Testing Department at the Royal Liverpool Hospital for her kind assistance with the JPD patients and preparation of this article. I would also like to express my gratitude to Dr J. L. Verbov, Consultant Dermatologist, and Professor Vickers, Professor of Dermatology, together with the staff of the Royal Liverpool Children's Hospitals, Myrtle Street and Alder Hey branches, for their cooperation in investigating and reporting their cases of JPD.

## REFERENCES

1. Silvers, S. H. and Glickman (1968). Atopy and eczema of the feet in children. *Am. J. Dis. Child.*, **116,** 400–401
2. Enta, T. (1972). Peridigital dermatitis in children. *Cutis*, **10,** 325–328
3. Möller, H. (1972). Atopic winter feet in children. *Acta Dermatovenereol.* (*Stockh.*), **52,** 401–405
4. Schultz, H. and Zachariae, H. (1972). The trafuril test in recurrent juvenile eczema of hands and feet. *Acta Dermatovenereol.* (*Stockh.*), **52,** 398–400
5. Mackie, R. M. and Husain, S. I. (1976). Juvenile plantar dermatosis: A new entity? *Clin. Exp. Dermatol.*, **1,** 253–260
6. Hambly, E. M. and Wilkinson D. S. (1978). Sur quelques formes atypiques d'eczema chez l'enfant. *Ann, Derm. Venereol.*, **105,** 369–371
7. Friis, B. (1973). Dermatitis plantaris sicca hos born. *Ugaskr. Laeg.*, **135,** 1466–1470
8. Maleville, J., Marsan, Ph., Coindre, M-Cl., Ducombs, G., Duboz, A., Taieb, A. and Guillet, G. (1984). Pulpite seche de l'avant-pied. *Annales de Pediatrie*, **31,** 291–294
9. Steck, W. D. (1983). Juvenile plantar dermatosis: 'The wet and dry foot syndrome'. *Cleveland Clin Q.*, **50,** 145–149
10. Gibson, W. B. (1963). Sweaty sock dermatitis. *Clin. Pediatr.*, **2,** 175–177
11. Graham, R. M., Verbov, J. L. and Vickers, C. F. H. (1987). Juvenile plantar dermatosis. *Clin. Exp. Dermatol.*, **12,** 468–469
12. Weston, J. A., Hawkins, K. and Weston, W. L. (1983). Foot dermatitis in children. *Pediatrics.*, **72,** 824–827
13. Van Dijk, E., Van Ketel, W. G., Neering, H., Nelemans, Th.G., Roeleveld, C. G. and Verburgh-Van Der Zwan, N. (1978). Juvenile plantaire dermatose; een nieuw ziektebeeld? *Ned. T. Geneesk.*, **122,** 223–228
14. Ashton, E. E., Russell Jones, R. and Griffiths A. (1985). Juvenile plantar dermatosis. *Arch. Dermatol.*, **121,** 225–228
15. Lim, K. B., Tan, T. and Rajan, V. S. (1986). Dermatitis palmaris sicca a distinctive pattern of hand eczema. *Clin. Exp. Dermatol.*, **11,** 553–559
16. Verbov, J. (1978). Atopic dermatitis and the forefoot. *Br. Med. J.*, **2,** 962
17. Czarnecki, D. B., Cowen, P. S. and Connors, T. J. (1981). Juvenile plantar dermatosis in an adult. *Br J. Dermatol.*, **104,** 599–600
18. Mackie, R. M. (1982). Juvenile plantar dermatosis. *Semin. Dermatol.*, **1,** 67–71
19. Young E. (1986). Forefoot eczema–further studies and a review. *Clin. Exp. Derm.*, **11,** 523–528
20. Stankler. L. (1978). Juvenile plantar dermatosis in identical twins. *Br. J. Dermatol.*, **99,** 585
21. Moorthy, T. T. and Rajan, V. S. (1984). Juvenile plantar dermatosis in Singapore. *Int. J. Dermatol.*, **23,** 476–479
22. Ashton, R. E. and Griffiths, W. A. D. (1986). Studies on sweating and bacterial

ecology in juvenile plantar dermatosis. *Clin. Exp. Dermatol.*, **11,** 535–542
23. Molokhia, M. (1981). Uninvolved foot areas sweat more. Symposium: Juvenile plantar dermatitis, King's College Cambridge, *Symposium Bulletin*, Sept. 1981.
24. Shrank, A. B. (1978). The aetiology of juvenile plantar dermatosis. *Br. J. Dermatol.*, **100,** 641–648.
25. Verbov, J. (1978). Atopic eczema localised to the forefoot – an unrecognised entity. *Practitioner*, **220,** 465–466
26. Hole, L. G. (1973). Sweat disposal from footwear and health and hygiene of foot skin. *J. Soc. Cosmet. Chem.*, **24,** 43–63
27. Hole, G. L. (1981). Sweat accumulation in footwear and juvenile plantar dermatosis. Symposium: Juvenile plantar dermatosis. King's College Cambridge. *Symposium Bulletin*, Sept. 1981.
28. Kint, A., Van Hecke, E. and Leys, G. (1982). Dermatitis plantaris sicca. *Dermatologica*, **165,** 500–509
29. Stewart, W. M. (1971). "Digito pulpite keratosique et fissuraire" et retention sudorale. *Ann. Dermatol. Syphiligraphie*, **95,** 49–52
30. Sulzberger, M. B. and Harris, D. R. (1972). Miliarier and Anhidrosis. *Arch. Dermatol.*, **105,** 845–850
31. Levy, A., Hanau, D. and Foussereau, J. (1980). Contact dermatitis in children. *Contact Dermatitis.*, **6,** 260–262
32. Angelini, G. and Meneghini, C. L. (1977). Contact and bacterial allergy in children with atopic dermatitis. *Contact Dermatitis*, **3,** 163–174
33. Jones, S. K., English, J. S. C., Forsyth, A. and MacKie, R. M. (1987). Juvenile plantar dermatosis – an 8 year follow-up of 102 patients. *Clin Exp. Dermatol.*, **12,** 5–7
34. White, M. I., Milne, R. M. and Main, R. A. (1978). Juvenile plantar dermatosis: Further observations on the aetiology. *Clin. Exp. Dermatol.*, **3,** 218
35. Hanifin, J. M. (1978). Nike training shoe dermatitis. *Arch. Dermatol.*, **114,** 289
36. Ashton, R. E. and Griffiths, W. A. D. (1986). Juvenile plantar dermatosis – atopy or footwear? *Clin. Exp. Dermatol.*, **11,** 529–534
37. Medansky, R. S. and Handler, R. M. (1974). Treatment of eczematous eruptions – a double-blind study using a porous lubricating cream base. *Clin. Med.*, **81,** 27–28

# 5

# CUTANEOUS RESPONSES TO ARTHROPODS

*G. S. WALTON*

## INTRODUCTION

Cutaneous changes may be produced by arthropods feeding off, developing on, or attacking the skin; such changes may result from –

1. mechanical damage;
2. the deposition of irritant, cytotoxic or pharmacologically active substances;
3. the presence or deposition of potential allergens;
4. the stimulation of a persistent insect bite or foreign-body response;
5. the introduction of infective agents;

Mechanical damage is usually of minor importance, unless associated with heavy infestation of *Demodex folliculorum*, *Tunga penetrans*, myiasis or the overwhelming attacks of certain flying insects.

Cutaneous changes always follow the deposition of the irritant, cytotoxic and pharmacologically active substances contained within the venoms of such insects as bees, wasps, hornets and scorpions.

Conversely, many arthropods living on or feeding off the skin initially do so without producing any obvious evidence of discomfort or cutaneous change, as they produce a minimum of mechanical damage and they or their secretions are devoid of noxious material. Such arthropods may, however, contain or secrete a number of substances that are potential allergens, and to which individuals may become sensitized after a variable period of either continuous or repeated exposure. Continuing or subsequent exposure to the relevant allergen will then result in the production of either an immediate anaphylactic and/or a delayed allergic response.

Immediate reactions to the secretions of biting insects are often typified by the appearance of a local cutaneous urticarial lesion shortly after challenge that subsides several hours later unless the area is traumatized. On rare occasions, following the bite of certain insects, this response may be accompanied by a more profound response – typified by a more generalized urticaria, angio-oedema, or generalized anaphylaxis often leading, in the absence of immediate treatment, to death.

Initiation of a delayed allergic response to the secretions of biting insects often precedes the development of the immediate type of allergic response in many individuals. A delayed allergic response is frequently characterized by a inflammatory nodule and accompanied by pain and/or irritation – the response only being noted after a delay of several hours following challenge. Once established, it persists for 5 to 8 days, or for a longer period if it is rubbed or if a similar challenge occurs elsewhere on the skin, when not only will a similar lesion occur at the second site, but there will be recurrence of inflammation over the original area. Thus, patients who have been subjected to continuous or intermittent attack over a period of several days or weeks often present with large numbers of cutaneous lesions.

On rare occasions, a delayed systemic response may occur in subjects, producing a local delayed hypersensitivity reaction – typified by Schönlein–Henoch purpura and/or massive haemorrhagic changes involving internal organs, which again can prove lethal.

Occasionally, following insect bites or infestation, an irritant nodule is produced that persists for many months. Histologically, there may be evidence of pseudocarcinomatous hyperplasia together with a dense inflammatory infiltrate within the dermis, containing eosinophils, plasma cells, lymphocytes and histiocytes. The factors involved in the production of this response are poorly understood and remain a matter for conjecture, but certain individuals appear to be prone to developing this type of response when infested with or attacked by a particular arthropod.

Bacterial, viral, parasitic or fungal infections may always present as possible complications in arthropod infestation.

The diagnosis of arthropod-induced skin disease can present a clinical challenge. However, detailed examination of the type and distribution of lesions, linked with close investigation of the patient's environment and all circumstantial evidence, can prove rewarding and form the basis for further investigations, leading to the isolation and identification of the relevant arthropod. A detailed knowledge of the habitat, life-cycle, nutritional requirements and survival of a given arthropod is essential, and these factors will be discussed in relation to those arthropods that are commonly responsible for disease in man.

## HYMENOPTERA

Members of this very large order of insects, which contains bees, wasps, hornets, yellow jackets and ants, do not feed off man, but if provoked may attack, inoculating their venom deep into the skin.

The chemical constitution of Hymenoptera venom is complex and subject to familial and species variation. It contains both antigenic material and pharmacologically active agents.

The venom of some bees contains histamine, lecithinase and cholinesterase. The venom of some species of wasp contains histamine, 5-hydroxytryptamine and bradykinin, whilst European hornet venom contains histamine, 5-hydroxytryptamine and a kinin, and is a rich source of acetylcholine.

Despite these variations, inoculation of venom into the skin produces an immediate burning sensation, accompanied by local hyperaemia and swelling. Systemic collapse may occur following multiple stings or when the face or mucous membranes are attacked.

If sensitized individuals are attacked, a more severe local reaction occurs. Also, in such individuals there is an increased possibility of generalized anaphylaxis or serious delayed allergic reactions, Hymenoptera having been responsible for more fatalities in the United States between 1950 and 1959 than poisonous snakes, spiders or other biting insects.

It is important to appreciate that bee-keepers may also react violently to the inhalation of bee antigens.

Recently, the efficacy of specific IgE, skin testing and the application of immunotherapy in the diagnosis and management of such patients has been seriously questioned.

Fortunately, linking the presenting lesions with members of this group of insects rarely presents a diagnostic problem, with the exception of multiple lesions noted on inhabitants of houses infested with either the small house wasp or certain species of ant.

## DIPTERA

Many insects included in this order are not only important vectors of human disease but also a frequent cause of cutaneous lesions in man.

*Mosquitoes* (*Culicidae*) are free-flying insects possessing a spherical head, elongated thorax, long legs and antennae, a wedge-shaped abdomen and long, narrow wings that flatten over the abdomen when at rest.

Their breeding requirements show marked species variation. Although the majority lay their eggs in or near water, temperature, acidity, alkalinity, salt concentration or the presence or absence of decaying vegetable matter can profoundly affect the capacity of a given species to inhabit any one area.

Environmental temperature can influence development. Lower temperatures can inhibit development, but the eggs of some species can resist cold and drying for a considerable time or can prolong the larval period for several months. Females of some species can hibernate in buildings or barns in cold weather or oestrovate in hot conditions until the next season.

Adults may fly several miles from their breeding sites to feed; they can also be transported several miles on the wind, or greater distances in vehicles or aeroplanes.

Males feed on nectar and fruits. The females require a blood meal before commencing egg laying. Feeding activity is higher in subdued evening light and at night, but the insects may be attracted by light and enter houses to rest or feed. During the day they tend to rest, unless disturbed.

The mechanisms by which mosquitoes are attracted to their host require further investigation – warmth, humidity, possibly carbon dioxide levels, dark clothing, lysine and certain aminoacids all appear to aid attraction. This attraction can be increased in anhidrotics by wetting the skin.

The salivary secretions of mosquitoes are non-irritant. In non-sensitized individuals, although a blood spot may mark the feeding site, no other reaction is usually seen.

Initially, sensitized individuals develop a delayed response, typified by the production of itchy papules that appear several hours after feeding has taken place and persist for several days. Later, such individuals may present with a papular urticarial, or on rare occasions a bullous, response, which appears very shortly following feeding and is followed by a delayed response over that area or areas. Following further attacks the delayed response may be lost and following repeated attacks the immediate response may finally disappear. Individuals who are subject to only very intermittent attack may remain sensitized for many years. Cross-sensitivity between the different salivary secretions of some species of mosquito does exist but is not complete, and requires further investigation.

Bite lesions are noted most frequently over exposed areas of the body.

Sufferers should be advised to avoid breeding areas and to curtail outside activities during the evening and early night in mosquito-ridden areas and to avoid shady areas at other times during the day; advice should also include closing lighted room windows and checking all rooms for the presence of mosquitoes before retiring for the night.

The skin may be protected by clothing or mosquito netting impregnated with an insect repellant if infested areas cannot be avoided. Mosquito netting over windows and/or beds is essential in some areas.

Fly repellants, such as dimethyl or dibutyl phthalate or diethyltoluamide appear to help in some but not all cases. It should be appreciated that these substances are often very short-acting and can damage plastics, including some spectacle frames.

On very rare occasions, more severe systemic responses have been noted in association with this group of insects, but their most serious role is as a vector of other diseases.

*Gnats, midges, punkies or 'no-see-ums'* (*Ceratopogonidae*) are minute free-flying insects with the thorax humped over the head, possessing hair covered wings that are flattened over the thorax at rest. Their eggs are laid and develop in water.

The females of some species requires a blood meal before egg laying commences. Adults are capable of travelling several miles from breeding sites.

Feeding takes place during the periods of subdued light in the early morning and evening, but the feeding period is extended on dull days, in shaded areas and around breeding grounds. It is unable to feed under windy conditions or in strong air currents.

Its size allows it to pass through normal mosquito netting.

The bite is usually non-irritant, but in hypersensitive patients it produces similar lesions to those noted in association with hypersensitivity to mosquito bites. Preventive measures are similar to those described for the latter, but insecticidal spraying of breeding areas can be of great value in eradicating a local problem.

*Black flies or buffalo gnats* (*Simuliidae*) are small insects similar in size to midges, but possessing a short piercing proboscis (which is used to slash the skin of its prey). The wings are broad and hairless and the body is covered with short golden or silver hairs.

They breed in large numbers in fast-flowing streams or rivers and around such areas they often make conditions intolerable for both animals and man for many months of the year.

Initially, their bites may be painless and the only indication may be the presence of blood oozing from the sites they attack – which are usually confined to exposed areas of the body. Later, following sensitization, immediate papular urticarial and/or delayed nodular lesions may be seen.

As these insects often congregate in very large numbers, cases of severe regionalized or generalized skin oedema leading to systemic collapse and death have been recorded both in animals and man, when they have become enveloped in swarms of these insects.

Feeding usually takes place in the early evening and it is advisable to avoid infested areas at that time.

As these insects tend to alight on clothing prior to feeding, it is essential that all areas of the body are protected, when going into or near infested areas. It is essential that any gaps in clothing around the neck, wrists and legs are obliterated. Fine gauge netting suspended over the face and the use of gloves are of value. Dark-coloured clothing appears to attract this family of insects. Insect repellants are of little value.

Spraying breeding sites with insecticides has been successful, but is ecologically unacceptable in most cases.

*Sandflies or 'owl midges'* (*Psychodidae*) are small moth-like flying insects usually under 5 mm in length, possessing hair-covered wings and bodies, and beard-like antennae. The wings are held roof-like over the body at rest. Eggs are laid in and develop in dark moist areas in crevices, under stones or in dense vegetation, when the temperature is above 15°C. The larvae feed on dried vegetation or faecal material.

The females of some species are blood sucking, feeding at night and hiding during the day. They are weak fliers but can get through mosquito netting and when hungry will search for any openings in doors, windows or clothing to gain access to their prey.

Initially, patients often present with papular urticarial lesions or itchy nodules with superficial crusting and involving exposed areas of the body, such as the volar areas of the wrists, dorsal areas of the hands, the legs, dorsal areas of the feet and the face. Vesicle formation may also occur in some individuals.

Prevention can present a major problem for patients sleeping in the open or under canvas in infested areas.

*Horse flies or breeze flies* (*Tabanidae*) are large, often brown-coloured insects with large eyes and large powerful hairless veined wings that are held in a divergent position over the body at rest. They breed near water in muddy areas. They love sunlight and are daytime feeders, usually attacking several exposed areas of the body on each occasion. They produce painful punctate lesions with haemorrhagic centres and varying degrees of oedema.

Insect repellants are of little value, but the problem can usually be reduced by vigilance and avoiding areas in or around breeding sites. It should be appreciated that if these insects are disturbed whilst resting, they invariably start to feed in daylight hours.

*Stable flies* (*Stomoxys*) are similar in appearance to the house fly, but the thorax is grey with four dark longitudinal bars. The abdomen is plumper and has three dark spots on both the second and third segments. Both male and female flies are blood suckers. Feeding takes place in daylight and lasts for several minutes at any one time and often involves moving to a number of different sites.

Although in inclement weather they may enter buildings, they usually rest on the exposed areas of buildings or similar sites.

After ingesting several blood meals, the female lays batches of eggs in damp, decaying vegetable matter, urine-stained hay and straw, or manure. Development through larval and pupal stages to adulthood takes four to five weeks in mild weather. Adults live for a similar period.

Feeding is often accompanied by a delayed but painful sensation and the production of a raised punctate urticarial weal from which a small amount of blood may ooze.

Avoidance of breeding localities is advised; where this is not possible, an attempt should be made to remove and destroy breeding material.

*The pigeon fly* (*Pseudolynchia*) is a small dark brown fly 6 mm long that occasionally infests pigeons and wild birds. The larvae develop in cracks and crevices or nesting material. Occasionally this blood-sucking fly can be responsible for the production of papular urticarial lesions on people handling infested birds or working in infested pigeon lofts, the lesions most frequently involving the face, arms and hands.

The fly can be difficult to find, but fumigation of infested buildings and the use of pyrethrum or derris on infested birds produces good results.

*Tsetse flies* (*Glossina*), apart from their role as vectors of disease, produce similar cutaneous changes to those noted in association with *Stomoxys*, but do not occur, and are of no importance, outside the continent of Africa. They and many other insects that are capable of feeding off, invading, or producing myiasis in previously damaged skin, are excluded from discussion in this chapter.

## APHANIPTERA

*Fleas* (*Siphonaptera*) are, after free-flying insects, probably one of the most common causes of cutaneous lesions in man in many parts of the world. Over 1600 species of flea have been identified and over 60 species occur in the UK.

Fleas, despite often being designated to a specific host (e.g. cat flea, dog flea, human flea), are not host-specific, and when hungry will feed off a variety of hosts.

These small brown insects are fast-moving, capable of jumping considerable distances (in relation to their size), and when hungry have a great capacity for hunting down a suitable host. Although they may remain for some time in the coat of animals, in man they drop off and disappear into clothing or their surroundings having fed.

The female flea requires a blood meal before commencing egg laying. If the temperaure is above 55°F and climatic conditions are favourable, she may lay up to 500 eggs in her lifetime. Under favourable conditions the egg will hatch out within a few days to produce a small caterpillar-like larva that, having ingested minute amounts of dried blood, faeces or organic matter, retires into carpeting, a crevice (or in hot climates soil or sand), spins a cocoon and pupates. In the pupal form it can survive for several months, withstanding low temperatures and arid conditions. Finally it will emerge, frequently as the result of being stimulated by either movement or mechanical vibration, as a fit, active and hungry adult.

Flea saliva is non-irritant and initially flea bites are asymptomatic; however, following repeated challenge, hypersensitivity develops to one of the antigenic fractions it contains (which are thought to be haptenic in nature and require to be linked to elements of the skin before reaching full antigenicity).

Once sensitization has occurred, an immediate papular urticarial response and/or a delayed nodular response will be produced over the bite site, as described previously. Systemic changes rarely occur, but angio-oedema can be a complication in certain individuals and, as with bites of flying insects, blister formation is possible. Hyposensitization can occur following repeated or prolonged infestation.

Fleas, unlike free-flying insects, produce most lesions under clothing and on the upper leg. As they feed several times on the one occasion, patients often present with a number of lesions showing a clumped or linear pattern. In long-standing cases of persistent infestation, patients displaying a delayed response may present with hundreds of lesions widely distributed over the body.

In congested communities possessing low standards of hygiene, flea infestations may be entirely supported by the human population. In suburban areas, enjoying low population densities and a high standard of hygiene, maintenance of the flea population is often dependent upon the family dogs and cats, who are often responsible for its introduction and help to support it. On rare occasions, flea infestation in premises can be derived from wild or domestic birds or rodents inhabiting the premises.

In the family situation, usually one or two members of a group present with lesions (often the younger members), despite all having been attacked, and on many occasions the family pets show no evidence of irritation or skin changes.

Diagnosis can present difficulties. In cases of heavy infestation, adult fleas or flea debris may be found in clothing or bedding. In light infestations, despite the presence of many cutaneous lesions, evidence is sometimes difficult to find. Animal-derived infestations require the microscopical examination of coat grooming and/or the contents of baskets and blankets.

When infestation is light or intermittent and hygiene is good, palliative treatment of lesions may suffice. In cases of heavy infestation and where hygiene is poor, the property should be thoroughly cleaned and the premises fumigated or fogged.

In tropical areas it may be necessary to spray the ground around the property.

Animal-based infestations are often best combated by seeking veterinary treatment of the family pet using insecticidal baths, powders, sprays or collars, or even systemic treatment, with the aim not only of destroying the animal's infestation, but also to make it into an animated flea trap as an aid to stopping reinfestation.

*The stick fast flea* (*Tunga penetrans*), a resident in many tropical areas of the world, presents a different problem. The female, after feeding and copulation, burrows deep into the dermis of the feet and toes and less frequently the perianal skin, scrotum, face or other parts of the body.

In the early stages of infestation in animals and man, the site of penetration appears as a raised nodule with a black centre. At this stage it may be opened and the parasite exposed and expelled.

Once established the flea starts to feed, swells, commences to ovulate and defecate, producing a large pustular swelling, which may coalesce with any adjacent lesions forming large plaques possessing a honeycomb appearance and leading possibly to cellulitis, septicaemia, lymphangitis, clostridial infection or just areas of slow-healing ulceration.

As this flea normally inhabits dry sand or soil in and around human and animal accommodation, steps must be taken to eliminate infestation from these areas using parasiticidal sprays. Advice should be given on hygiene and the constant wearing of shoes and clothing, and on life style.

## CIMICIDAE

*Bedbugs and related species* (*Cimicidae*) are small, oval, yellow to dark-brown insects (5 mm × 3 mm), flattened dorsoventrally and possessing vestigial wings. They can infest man, animals and birds.

The female lays 100–200 eggs within crevices over a period of several days to weeks, depending on the environmental temperature. On hatching, larvae are produced that, after five nymphal stages, reach maturity in 2 to 5 months. Adults can survive in infested premises for over a year without food.

It is a nocturnal feeder, emerging after dark from nooks and crevices, attracted by the warmth of human, avian or animal bodies to feed. Despite its size, it is capable of travelling considerable distances, through roof spaces or between buildings or apartments. It can be transported in furniture, luggage or on vermin to new areas. It is a greedy feeder, often attacking the skin in several places during one night.

The bite is initially painless and does not waken the quarry. Urticarial lesions possessing a punctate centre, often capped with a blood spot, result in many cases. Nodular reaction may occur and bullous lesions may also be noted in some individuals. Irritation can be intense and can be accompanied by a general malaise.

In the UK, lesions are most frequently encountered over the neck, shoulders, arms and hands. They are easily confused with responses to free-flying insects, but the legs are rarely involved.

In hot climates and with persistent infestation, the distribution of lesions is more widespread and less characteristic.

Examination of the patient is rarely rewarding, but microscopical examination of brushings obtained from nooks, crevices, picture rails, or from behind wallpaper may reveal the insect. Alternatively, if the patient is aroused two hours before daybreak and bed linen and night attire are quickly removed and shaken into a plastic bag and the collected contents then examined, a diagnosis can often be reached.

Thorough cleaning of the premises, including cupboards, etc., followed by fumigation and the eradication of vermin is essential, together with a close study of surrounding habitations.

## SARCOPTIFORMES

*Sarcoptiforme mites* are a very large group, some of which are parasitic on man, animals, birds or other creatures. The latter tend to be host specific, spending their entire existence on or in the skin, where they complete their life cycle.

The pattern of cutaneous changes associated with *Sarcoptes scabiei hominis* has been the subject of numerous papers and will not be discussed.

Animal and bird mange mites tend to be host specific, producing hyperaemia, scaling and irritation in the skin of their definitive host. Survival away from the definitive host is usually short-lived. Many can survive for several days on man, but are unable to burrow or complete their life cycle.

However, individuals who repeatedly come into contact with one of these ectoparasites by continually handling infested animals or birds, or infested debris, may, after a variable period, become sensitized to such mites; further contact results in the production of a skin response. This presents as areas of either pin-point eruptions or fiery red papules. Irritation is severe and can become intolerable should the subject start to sweat or the skin be heated.

Fortunately, infested animals or birds will always show some evidence of cutaneous change and if a diagnosis is to be achieved, possible sources of infestation must be investigated.

Chorioptic mange in horses is common in the winter months, causing an irritant scaling reaction involving the legs and occasionally the face and neck, lesions often resolving in the summer. On rare occasions, horse handlers may suffer from skin changes involving the lower arm and sides of the neck and face. Equine sarcoptic and psoroptic mange infestations are rare, but during the Great War 'cavalry man's itch' was common as a result of contact with these mites and produced widespread lesions on the legs and elsewhere on the body.

Sarcoptic and psoroptic mange present a problem in some dairy and beef units, causing irritant scaly lesions over wide areas of the bovine skin. Cowmen working with such animals may develop skin lesions on the arms, sides of the face and neck. Lesions are frequently found round waist-bands where infested scale tends to lodge. Occasionally, the cowman may show no lesions, but where he takes infested material into the farm house, lesions may be noted in other members of the family. Similar lesions may be produced by contact with cattle suffering from chorioptic mange, which, during the winter, produces in those animals a milder scaling reaction involving the tail, head and occasionally the neck.

Mange in sheep is notifiable in the UK and it is unlikely that it has the opportunity to produce lesions on man.

Sarcoptic mange has been common in pigs, producing a scaling reaction of varying severity over the back and other parts of the body and causing pigman's itch – a thickened irritant scaly reaction, in chronic cases involving the lower arm.

Sarcoptic mange in the dog occurs sporadically. It causes irritation, hyperaemia and scaling over the ear flaps, face, limbs and, in puppies, can become generalized. Individual members of the family handling infested animals may present with lesions on the lower arms (rarely the hands), face, neck and less frequently the legs. More generalized lesions occur if the animal shares the owners' bed. Noteadric mange is now rare in the cat, but will produce a similar pattern of lesions to that seen in the dog. Ear mange (Otodectes) in the dog and cat occasionally causes small areas of cutaneous change on the hands, arms or face of human contacts.

The role of canine *Demodex* infestation is debatable, but it has been incriminated in the production of human lesions.

Rabbits, guinea-pigs, mice, rats and other rodents all have their own species of mange mites and can be responsible for the production of lesions on the arms of staff who work in commercial or experimental establishments. Conversely, the lesions produced in children possessing these types of pets often have a bizarre distribution and pattern, which can involve any part of the body, such as around the waistband or involving the skin beneath a pocket area.

*Cnemidocoptes* infestation in birds affect the beak and legs; lesions seen in bird fanciers most frequently involve the hands, wrists and sides of the face.

Isolation of mites from human lesions is usually unsuccessful.

Diagnosis of mange in animals and birds rests on clinical examination of the relevant animals or birds, and is confirmed by microscopical examination of their skin debris. Provided the source of infestation is either eliminated or treated successfully, lesions in man will usually resolve spontaneously within 10 to 14 days; this period may be reduced slightly if a mild acaricide is used.

## PHTHIRAPTERA

*Louse infestation* (*pediculosis*) in man has been the subject of numerous articles and will not be discussed. Louse infestations may occur in all species of domestic animal and bird. Lice are host specific and although animal and bird lice may be found on man occasionally, they die rapidly and are not known to produce cutaneous changes.

## CHEYLETIELLA

*Fur mites (Cheyletiella)* are small ectoparasites (0.4 mm long), possessing a shield-shaped body, well developed hooked palps, and feathered legs with combed tarsi. A number of species have been recognized living on animals and birds; those found on the rabbit, cat and dog are of particular importance in human skin disease.

Although they can produce irritation and heavy coat scaling, sometimes described as creeping dandruff, many animals carry heavy infestations without any evidence of coat or skin changes and some have, in fact, won major shows because of their apparent excellent condition!

Severe skin changes can be produced by this mite in humans involved with infested animals – changes typified by grouped, raised erythematous nodules with necrotic centres that are invariably situated on the trunk or underclothing, give a burning sensation when rubbed and are otherwise extremely irritant, persisting for several weeks in some cases.

Frequently, only one or two members of a family or group handling infested animals is affected at one time.

Attempted isolation of the mite from the patient or clothing is usually disappointing, but microscopical examination of animal skin debris is rewarding. Palliative treatment of human lesions is indicated. Appropriate parasiticidal treatment of all infested animals is easily carried out, and when done properly is very successful.

## ACARINA

*Fowl mites (Dermanyssidae)* are small spider-like mites (1–1.5 mm long), possessing a large dorsal shield and well-developed legs. Two species are of particular importance – the red fowl mite (*Dermannyssus gallinae*) and the northern fowl mite (*Ornithonyssus sylvarium*). Their definitive hosts are poultry, cage birds, wild birds and occasionally rodents.

They are fast-moving and nocturnal, resting in crevices during the day, but capable of moving great distances through buildings and ventilation shafts at night.

The female mite, after a blood meal, commences to lay eggs in or near nest sites or in convenient crevices. The life cycle is completed rapidly, usually within 7 to 14 days, and this can lead to the appearance of massive infestations inside buildings over a very short period of time. Mites can survive without food for up to 34 weeks (i.e. from one bird-nesting season to the next). Infestation can be carried on birds from one site to another in succeeding years.

Human infestation results either from working with infested poultry or cage birds, or from mites infesting the nests of wild birds (e.g. sparrows, starlings, pigeons) situated in the eaves, roof spaces or gutters of houses, offices, hostels or hospitals.

The mite produces discrete itchy, inflammatory, and sometimes persistent, nodules on any part of the body.

Similar responses may also be seen in association with the tropical rat mite (*Ornithonyssus bacoti*), the tropical fowl mite (*Ornithonyssus bursa*), the house mouse mite (*Allodermanyssus sanguineus*), and also the bugs *Cimex oeciacus* (which has been found in swallows' nests) and *Haematosiphon inodora* (a common parasite of birds and poultry in parts of the Americas).

Examination of clothing is disappointing. The best results are achieved by embarking on a thorough search of all relevant buildings and their surroundings, appreciating that the severest cutaneous changes in man often occur after the definitive host has either been destroyed or has vacated the premises.

Destruction of all nests and nesting material is essential, and very thorough cleaning, followed by fumigation or fogging, is necessary to achieve success. In some outbreaks, this may need to be carried out on several occasions.

## IXODOIDEA

*Ticks (Ixodoidae)* are large, leathery mites of which there is a very large number of species, each showing variations in morphology, lifestyle, habitat and geographical distribution.

They have been classified into several families. The Ixodidae (hard ticks) and the Argasidae (soft ticks) are of profound importance – not only as they surpass all other arthropods in their capacity to transmit infectious diseases to animals and man, but also because it is essential that the larvae, nymphs and adults obtain a blood meal by attaching to the skin of a suitable host before either the life cycle progresses or egg laying commences.

*Ixodes ricinus (The castor bean or sheep tick)* is the commonest species found in the UK, where it feeds principally on cattle, sheep and wild mammals. There it predominates on hill and marginal land. In other countries with wetter climates it may be found on lower pastures.

The engorged female tick can lay several thousand eggs on the ground or in undergrowth, and these hatch out to produce small (1 mm) six-legged larvae, which, after a blood meal, moult in the ground to form eight-legged nymphs that, in turn, after another blood meal, moult on the ground to produce either adult males (2–3 mm) or adult females (up to 1 cm) that continue the cycle after a blood meal.

Feeding activity is most marked in the spring (March–June) or in the spring and early autumn (late August–November), depending on the region. At such times, the parasite migrates to the surface of vegetation or the tips of leaves or blades of grass to be in a strategic position for transferring onto any suitable passing host – which can be man.

A second tick, *Dermacentor reticulatus*, is also found in southern Britain. It tends to mimic *Ixodes ricinus*, but its larvae and nymphs tend to be more active in July and August, parasitizing small mammals predominantly. This parasite frequently occurs in wooded areas, where *Haemaphysalis punctata* may also occur.

In London and the Home Counties and in and around other conurbations, *Ixodes hexagonus* (the hedgehog tick) can attack man. Eggs are laid in nests, burrows, undergrowth, garden sheds, etc. It is often associated with hedgehogs, foxes, badgers, stoats and small mammals.

*Ixodes canisuga* (the British dog tick) is now very rare, but was found in and around country hunt and dog kennels. Similarly, bird ticks occur very infrequently in the UK.

In the UK the most frequent sites of attachment in man are in the legs, feet and less often the arms, neck and scalp. Initially, attachment causes no discomfort and often larval and nymphal infestations go unnoticed as the parasites have fed and detached before any discomfort and the appearance of urticarial or nodular lesions with pinpoint centres on the host.

Infestation with adult ticks is often, in the early stages, misdiagnosed by the patient as a small painless growth – symptoms of pain and/or irritation, when they occur, only becoming obvious after the parasite has been present for several days.

Sensitized individuals may present with an area of marked skin oedema and/or erythema surrounding the engorging parasite. After the parasite has been removed or dropped off, a central area of necrotic ulceration or granulation is left, which remains extremely pruritic and is slow to heal or may develop into a persistent insect bite response.

Hair loss may occur, over and around scalp lesions.

On rare occasions a severe local erythematous halo may develop, with an icteric inner ring, which slowly enlarges peripherally and can reach a considerable size before fading (erythema chronicum migrans).

Systemic symptoms of malaise or pyrexia may accompany infestation and tick paralysis can be a serious problem associated with certain species of tick in some parts of the world.

Removal of adult ticks can be very difficult, with the ever-present danger of leaving the mouth parts still embedded. Insecticides should not be used. Immersing the parasite in benzene, chloroform, essential oils or tobacco juice is often successful, but it takes time for the parasite to disengage and this must not be hurried. Palliative treatment and sometimes the use of antibiotics are indicated.

## FORAGE MITES, KISSING BUGS, THRIPS

*Forage mites* is a loose term that may be used to describe a very large and assorted group of arthropods living in vegetation, vegetable matter and/or stored food. They vary greatly in conformation and size, being either macroscopic or microscopic. They can be either predators, feeding on other insects or mites, or vegetarian.

Knowledge of the 'forage mite' species that are capable of producing human cutaneous disease is very incomplete and the literature is, in part, confusing owing to many mites having several synonyms and to some lack of universal agreement on their classification. Despite such shortcomings, the larval or adult forms of some species of 'forage mite' are, without doubt, capable of producing skin irritation or stimulating cutaneous allergic responses in man.

It is certain that some free-living sarcoptiform (e.g. *Tyroglyphus longoir*, *Tyroglyphus casei*, *Tyrophagus putrescentiae*, *Calophagus krameri* and possibly *Acurus siro*) and the trombidiform (e.g. *Pyemotes ventricosus*) mites can be responsible for cutaneous reactions in man. Less frequently, severe reactions can be encountered associated with some of the larger free-living insects, such as members of the Reduviidae (kissing bugs) and some species of *Thysanoptera* (thrips).

The appearance and distribution of lesions is often bizarre, being influenced by the type and degree of exposure, the arthropod concerned and the host's response.

Patients with forage mite infestation may present with closely grouped pinpoint inflammatory lesions, closely grouped or widely distributed erythematous nodules or papular urticarial lesions, urticarial plaques, bullous eruptions, or other erythematous eruptions. When investigations have negated the possibility of other arthropod involvement, forage mites should always be considered.

It is essential that detailed information is obtained on the patient's occupation, leisure activities and home environment, and of any concurrent cutaneous responses in other members of the family or associates.

Patients working in flour mills, bakeries, animal feed merchants or similar establishments may present with extremely irritant patchy lesions involving the arms, head, neck and/or chest and waist-band areas; less frequently, the legs may be involved. On many occasions only one member of staff is affected.

In the majority of cases, sarcoptiform or trombidiform mites are responsible. A detailed microscopical examination of debris collected from working clothes, and if this fails from the works' premises, is required to confirm diagnosis. Palliative treatment is necessary to make life bearable.

This type of infestation is often impossible to combat, as food materials are involved; and if full protective clothing cannot be worn, a change of occupation may be required.

Similar lesions may occur in people working in horticulture and in glass-houses. Fumigation of infested buildings is possible and successful, as is redeployment of the patient elsewhere in the same establishment.

Outbreaks of skin lesions associated with the handling of infected cargoes may be seen in dockers and warehousemen. They often have a similar distribution to those described earlier and can be produced by a large variety of arthropods. Spontaneous improvement often follows when the cargo is dispersed, but cleaning and fumigation of premises may be required to prevent re-establishment of infestation.

Farm workers may suffer severe eruptions after handling infested cereals, straw or hay, or by working in, near or under rooms containing infested material; infestation in such material often persists for several years in barns, hay lofts, etc.

The lesions can appear on any part of the body. In some cases, particularly when *Psorogates* is responsible, several workers will show lesions and, particularly in stables, animals will also present with cutaneous lesions and severe irritation.

Farmers working in fields or hedgerows and members of the general public spending time in the countryside during the summer months may also become infested with sarcoptiform or trombidiform mites, lesions most frequently occurring on the legs and arms. Infrequently in the UK, a large, painful, raised swelling may be produced following the attack of *Reduvius personatus* (kissing bug), which in very limited areas infests hedgerows and woods, principally preying on other insects. In other parts of the world, similar species can enter houses and cause more serious problems.

A particular problem on some hill and marginal land in the UK is created by the harvest mite (*Trombicula autumnali*), the six-legged larval form of which attacks warm blooded mammals. It is a small insect, just visible to the naked eye and often has the appearance of red pepper.

The larvae hatch out in late August in southern counties, but in northern England, Wales and Scotland hatching is delayed until towards the end of September. The mites remain active for 5 to 6 weeks and at that time are capable of attaching themselves to exposed areas of skin in very large numbers. A severe irritating, pimply, inflammatory reaction results in most, but not all, individuals. Lesions are most frequently noted on the ankles and legs, but may occur elsewhere on the body – the axillae and groin are favourite sites if the sufferer has lain down or sat on infested ground. Palliative treatment is advised, the reaction often taking over a week to resolve. Avoidance of infested areas during the times of larval activity is necessary; if this is not possible, protective clothing should be worn. Applications of dimethyl phthalate or other insect repellants are also of help.

Forage mite infestations involving house plants are becoming an increasing problem. They are non-seasonal and may affect one or more members of a family and/or the family pet. The lesions may occur anywhere on the body and take the form of those previously described. They can be so widespread and irritating that systemic therapy is required.

Diagnosis requires the microscopical examination of plant debris, obtained by shaking or tapping the foliage of the plants onto a piece of paper or plastic.

Removal of infested plants, or the repeated use of insecticidal sprays, is essential, after which the occurrence of lesions will slowly wane over a period of 2 to 3 weeks.

## LEPIDOPTERA AND COLEOPTERA

The caterpillars of certain species of moth (Lepidoptera) are covered in venomous hairs. In southern and south-eastern England during the summer, the caterpillars of the Browntail moth (*Nygmia phaeorrhoea*) may be found browsing on vegetation. If they are handled or inadvertently come into direct contact with the skin, an extremely painful irritant rash is produced that may require palliative treatment. On rare occasions a similar reaction may be produced to the caterpillars of some species of Gypsy moth.

In other parts of the world, caterpillar dermatitis can present a more serious problem and may also cause systemic illness in some individuals.

Amongst the very large number of species of beetle (Coleoptera), one family – the oil and blister beetles (Meloidae) – are of medical importance, as their blood and genital organs contain cantharidin.

At least twelve species of this family occur in the UK. They vary markedly in size, shape and life-cycle, but should they inadvertently be crushed against the skin, a severe blistering reaction will ensue.

## FURTHER READING

1. Arthur, D.R. (1962). *Ticks and Disease*. (Oxford: Pergamon Press)
2. Barnard, J.H. (1967). Allergic and pathologic findings in 50 insect-sting fatalities. *J. Allergy*, **40,** 107–114
3. Benjamini, E., Feingold, B.F. and Kartman, L. (1960). Antigenic properties of the oral secretion of fleas. *Nature*, **188,** 959–960
4. Derbes, V.J. (1976). Injurious effects in man induced by animals. In Demis, D.J.,

Dobson, R.L. and McGuire, J. (eds.) *Clinical Dermatology*, Vol. 4 (New York: Harper & Row)
5. Evans, G.O.J., Sheals, J.G. and MacFarlane, D. (1961). *The Terrestrial Acari of the British Isles: An Introduction to their Morphology, Biology and Classification.* (London: British Museum)
6. Fallis, A.M. (1964). Feeding and related behaviour of female simuliidae (Diptera). *Exp. Parasit.*, **15,** 439–470
7. Flynn, R.J. (1973). *Parasites of Laboratory Animals*, pp. 337–492. (Ames: Iowa State University Press)
8. Gething, M.A. (1973). Cheyletiella infestation in small animals. *Vet. Bull. (Weybridge)*, **43** (2), 63–67
9. Hewitt, M., Walton, G.S. and Waterhouse, M. (1971). Pet infestations and human skin lesions. *Brit. J. Dermatol.*, **85,** 215–225
10. Hughes, A.M. (1961). The mites of stored food. *Tech. Bull.*, 9 (London: HMSO)
11. Jensen, O.M. (1962). Sudden death due to stings from bees and wasps. *Acta Pathol. Microbiol. Scand.*, **54,** 9–29
12. Kampelmacher, M.J. and Van Der Zwan, J.C. (1987). Provocation test with a living insect as a diagnostic tool in systemic reactions to bee and wasp venom: a prospective study with emphasis on the clinical aspects. *Clin. Allergy*, **17,** 317–327
13. Killby, V.A. and Silverman, P.H. (1967). Hypersensitivity reactions in man to specific mosquito bites. *Am. J. Trop. Med.*, **16,** 374–380
14. Loomis, E.C. (1962). External parasites. In Hofstad, M.S., Calnek, B.W., Helmbolt, C.F., Reid, W.M. and Yoder, H.W. Jr (eds.) *Diseases of Poultry*, **7,** pp. 667–704. (Ames: Iowa State University Press)
15. Marples, M.J. (1962). *Ecology of the Human Skin*, pp. 247–333. (Illinois: Charles C. Thomas)
16. McKeil, J.A. and West, A.S. (1961). Nature and causation of insect bite reactions. *Pediatr. Clin. N. Am.*, **8,** 295–317
17. Reisman, R.E. (1985). Stinging insect allergy: progress and problems (editorial). *J. Clin. Allergy*, **75,** 553–58
18. Shulman, S. (1968). Insect allergy: Biochemical and immunological analyses of the allergens. In Kallos, P. and Waksman, B.H. (eds.) *Progress in Allergy 12*, pp. 246–317 (Basel: S. Karger)
19. Taplin, D. (1986). Cutaneous infestations. In Vickers, C.F.H. (ed.) *Modern Management of Common Skin Diseases*, pp. 18–25. (Edinburgh: Churchill Livingstone)

# 6

# COMPUTER APPLICATIONS IN DERMATOLOGY

*A. Y. FINLAY*

## INTRODUCTION

Dermatologists not using computers are a dying breed. Every dermatologist in training that I know uses a word processor and many use their computer for other tasks. However, the impact that computer science has had on the dermatologist of the 1980s is minimal compared with the potential for change in the 1990s. The purpose of this chapter is to review some of the computer applications in dermatology that are already of practical importance and some that are of considerable potential interest. Word processing and the use of keeping a diagnostic index are discussed initially. The more exciting ability to access major databases is mentioned before a more detailed review of the controversial subject of computer diagnosis in dermatology. The important potential for computers in teaching and research is then stressed.

## WORD PROCESSING

The advantages of using a word processor in a department of dermatology, as in any other branch of medicine or business, are so obvious to those who use them that this topic may seem superfluous. All word processor users should skip this section. However, in a survey of members of the British Association of Dermatologists by their Computer Application Working Group in January, 1987, only 42%

of British dermatologists used a word processor. There are, therefore, even now in Britain and elsewhere many dermatologists who do not possess or use a word processor, and this section is directed at them.

After a letter or an article is typed on a word processor, mistakes can be corrected, alterations can be incorporated in the text, and the position of words, sentences and paragraphs can be altered without having to retype the whole letter or text again. The major advantage, therefore, of using a word processor instead of a typewriter is that the need for repetitive copy typing is abolished. The ease of altering mistakes means that even people with only very limited typing skills can produce perfect and professional-looking typed work.

In some systems, the word-processing software is permanently stored within the computer so that the computer acts as a 'dedicated' word processor. The use of a dedicated system is, however, not necessary, as virtually any computer with a printer can act as a word-processor with appropriate software. In either situation, once the word-processing software is in operation, text can be directly typed into the system on the computer keyboard and is instantly displayed on the screen. Any alterations needed can be carried out immediately, and the text can instantly be stored for retrieval at another time and can also be printed. On subsequent occasions the latest version of the text, or an earlier version if required, can instantly be recalled and further changes can be made.

The text can be printed very rapidly using a dot-matrix printer or more slowly using a daisywheel printer, which gives a range of typefaces identical to those available on a typewriter. The 24-pin dot-matrix printers now available make the quality of printing very close to that of a daisywheel, but in addition allow very flexible control over typeface output.

The flexibility of use of word processors soon makes them indispensable at any level in a dermatology department. One of the main tasks of most dermatology secretaries is to type clinic letters about patients to their general practitioners. Given equal availability of an electric typewriter and a word processor, a good typist may choose simply to use a typewriter for uncomplicated letters, but for any long or complicated letter in which there is an increased risk of mistakes being made or a risk of the dictating doctor changing his/her mind about a sentence or two, the word processor would always be chosen.

For any legal reports or administrative documents, the likelihood of errors needing correcting increases and so the word processor becomes more useful, and any work involving organization of meetings, teaching or writing articles is made much easier if a word processor is used.

If a 'standard letter' is used, the outline of the letter required can be stored and retrieved whenever necessary, and the specific patient information added. This produces a letter that is seemingly specific but in fact with little individual typing effort. Conversely, names and addresses can be stored and retrieved for use within letters or on envelopes, without having to copy type the name and address each time it is required.

The main arguments given by Shrank[1] for persuading dermatologists to introduce word processing facilities into their departments are: (1) Your letters will be more quickly produced, should contain no printing errors and will have a more professional look. (2) Your secretary will find the work more satisfying because it should be less tedious, and she produces a neat and attractive end-product. (3) By linking letter data with software for a Diagnostic Index, it becomes possible to keep efficiently a patient disease index. (4) Articles and reports will be more quickly prepared, and if you use the word processor yourself the text is more likely to express your meaning.

Once the facility for word processing is firmly established in a department, other uses of the computer soon become obvious. Immediate uses include keeping a file of one's curriculum vitae for easy updating. Using a simple database program, a record can be kept of references to other articles of interest and a file of reprints of articles held can be maintained[2].

## DATABASE

It is possible to run a dermatology service without attempting to keep any retrievable data. Such a service may provide excellent clinical advice, but is likely to be essentially a 'reactive' service and one in which little teaching or research takes place. Even the most uninterested dermatologist, however, will keep a note of the name of an extraordinary patient, illustrating the desire to keep at least some retrievable information. In contrast, many departments keep card-index files on all new patients and are therefore effectively able to access information on numbers of patients with different diagnoses, and are able to trace patients with a particular problem for research or teaching purposes.

There are obvious major advantages in storing departmental patient information on a computer. These include speed of access to information, and the ability to define and instantly find much more specific information. Stored information can be sorted by patient name, diagnosis or number, and there is great flexibility in the ability to handle data. One very useful feature of a computer-based patient diagnostic index is the facility to search for names or diagnoses without knowing the full name or even the correct spelling; a sequence of a few letters can be searched for. Individual entries can be identified so that, for instance, 'interesting patients' or 'patients who have agreed to attend a certain meeting' can be recalled rapidly.

There are a wide variety of commercially available database software packages, most of which are suitable for storing the data needed in a dermatology department. As the needs of many dermatologists are similar, the British Association of Dermatologists Computer Application Working Group has recently commissioned 'tailor-made' software, based on a commercial database package but with defined entry screens written to be appropriate for dermatology practice. The purpose of this software is for use as a department's main disease (diagnostic) index.

## Diagnostic index

The essential information that needs to be recorded in a department's computer database for a diagnostic index to be maximally valuable includes the following:

1. patient name and hospital number;
2. patient sex, age, date of birth;
3. patient address;
4. name of general practitioners (with address if appropriate);
5. diagnosis (primary and secondary): name and diagnostic code;
6. date of first consultation;

7. treatment or investigation codes;
8. name of dermatologist.

In addition, in a private office setting, the data stored could include details of billing and status of patients' accounts.

### *Disadvantages*

There are of course some disadvantages in storing all of a department's diagnostic information on a computer database. These range from legal considerations to risk of loss of data, but most potential disadvantages can be overcome with suitable planning.

When patient information is stored on a card system there is no legal obligation to register this information or to inform a patient that such data is specifically being kept. In contrast, in the United Kingdom, when data that can be identified with an individual is stored on computer, there is a legal obligation to register this database[3]. It then becomes possible for any patient or person about whom information is stored to have access to that information. In practice, in the short time that the law has existed, there has not been a rush of people checking their data; for practical purposes, once the legal obligations have been fulfilled the law should not affect the day-to-day use of a department's computer database. However, any operator should be aware of the possibility of any information stored being personally checked, and so information held should be accurate and sensitive information should be avoided.

Just as data held on cards is vulnerable to fire, to spilt coffee or to being dropped and disorganized, so data held on computer file is also potentially at risk. We are used to and can perhaps more easily accept the physical risks to a card system, but the unfamiliar risk of an even less predictable loss of computer information seems a disadvantage. Luckily, the ability to copy total information stored very rapidly means that backup copies of stored information can be taken regularly, so that if a disk holding large amounts of vital information does 'crash', there is always a recent copy available. In contrast, keeping a regular backup of written information, although physically possible with photocopiers, is so tedious as to be impractical with a large database.

Whereas a simple card-based diagnostic index is usually immediately understandable to all members of a dermatology department, some initial training will be needed for department members to use a computer-based index most effectively. In practice, however, the time involved is minimal, and general use of the departmental disease index unlikely to be retarded by reluctance to train.

## Clinical records

Databases of patient clinical information held on computer may, of course, be of practical value in the day-to-day running of a general or specialist dermatology clinic. Macfarlane *et al.*[4] have demonstrated the value of using a computer to handle the clinical results of a patch-testing clinic. Dooms-Goosens *et al.*[5] have also described the use of computer-assisted monitoring of a contact-dermatitis clinic. This system, known as CODEX, contains details of over 6000 pharmaceutical products that are applied to the skin, and details of over 7000 patients from three contact-dermatitis clinics in Belgium.

Where a series of investigations are carried out on a regular monthly or weekly basis, such as in the monitoring of patients taking long-term methotrexate, in a busy clinic the patient's notes tend to become cluttered with results. Although the results of investigations may be available, it can be very difficult to spot a slow trend of, say, falling haemoglobin or elevation of a liver enzyme. Simpson *et al.*[6] have described the use of a personal computer to store results in a clinic for monitoring patients with psoriasis taking methotrexate. This allows much more effective patient control, as sequential results can be displayed graphically, trends can be spotted and missing results or patient absences can be monitored more closely.

Similarly, in a PUVA clinic, record keeping, total UVA dosage and clinical status can all be monitored more effectively using a personal computer[7]. The record keeping in such clinics can primarily be carried out by a trained nurse, allowing more efficient and effective use of time by the physician, who can much more easily extract the relevant patient information.

## Hardware necessary

For a departmental database to work effectively, very large amounts of information need to be able to be stored. In any department with a throughput of, say, 6000 new patients each year, the storage and access facilities of a floppy disk system soon become overloaded. A hard-disk facility of at least 20 megabytes is necessary. If an IBM PC-compatible computer with 640 K RAM is chosen, the range of database software that can potentially be used is vast, and the cost of such a system, at less than £1000, is now dramatically less than even two or three years ago.

## Disease coding

If a new departmental disease index is being set up, it makes sense to use a coding system likely to be compatible with other departments. This allows direct comparison of data about different disease categories, and the use of an established code also considerably simplifies the setting up of a system, as questions of classification will usually have already been clarified. The current national disease coding index is based on the World Health Organization 'International Classification of Diseases'[8]. There are a number of flaws to this, the 9th revision, that are recognized by the authors and arise both from the parent classification's structural relationship with other specialities and also because it is now ten years old. The 10th revision is currently being produced, but unfortunately this will not be published until 1991; the use of the 9th revision with some local minor changes is a possible compromise until then.

## Database software

There are many database software systems available, some of which need more programming skill than others. The best known and most widely used has been dBASE III by Ashton-Tate. Although it remains one of the best and most flexible systems, it does need some skill in programming for non-standard applications. White[9] has described in detail how dBASE III may be used in a dermatology practice. Other systems, such as PC Promise or Reflex, may be easier and more friendly to use, and in fact there are other database systems available that use dBASE III but with a friendlier 'front-end'. This area changes so quickly that it is essential to check with current monthly computer journals before choosing a system.

## DERMATOLOGY INFORMATION

All dermatologists with the remotest flicker of interest in their speciality will at times be stimulated to search the literature for information about an interesting patient or a fascinating problem. For some, detailed literature searches are a routine part of academic life. Most of us fall between these two extremes and we are all familiar with searches of *Index Medicus*. Increasingly many are gaining the benefit of using computerized bibliographic information retrieval systems. There are several of these databases, which most major libraries will access and will provide a printout of a specific search. It is possible to carry out such a search on a personal computer at home using a modem attached to the telephone system. An example of a major computer base is MEDLARS, which is run by the National Library of Medicine in Bethesda[10]; software has been developed (GRATEFUL MED) to make personal access to this database more easy. There are other library databases, for example in Geneva, that can also be accessed by users in the United Kingdom; most databases are available for use internationally.

A recent review of communication software written to allow easier access to medical information databases such as DERM/INFONET[11] is of interest. DERM/INFONET is a group of dermatologic databases under the direction of the American Academy of Dermatology. Within DERM/INFONET it is possible to access a dermatology literature search DERM/MLS, treatment information DERM/RX and a drug database for dermatologists DERM/PHARM. DERM/RX gives therapeutic management options for several hundred skin diseases, and is constantly updated[12]. DERM/PHARM gives drug profiles on over 300 drugs used in dermatology[13]. The use of such databases is likely to increase rapidly over the coming years as more dermatologists discover their value.

## DIAGNOSIS

In 1964, when Norins suggested that computers could be used in dermatology for diagnosis, he commented that it would be very difficult for each physician to own a computer[14]. Twenty five years later, many physicians do own computers, but still practical computer aids to dermatology diagnosis have had very little impact. One of the problems in dermatology has been in quantifying the clinical information that we use, and this difficulty, which has delayed application of computer-aided diagnosis, is now being overcome both by new techniques of quantification and by newer methods of manipulating clinical information that do not rely on epidemiological data gathering.

In introducing the subject of computer-aided diagnosis, it must be admitted that there is a striking lack of enthusiasm about the concept amongst most practising clinical dermatologists. This reluctance to take the subject seriously may be due to a disbelief that the concept of computer diagnosis is possible in dermatology, or a sense that diagnostic skills are relatively unimportant in the subject. It may, however, be a response to a perceived major threat to professional status. This concern must be faced directly; the professional concept of a dermatologist is defined by the special ability of that physician to make a diagnosis, to advise on management and to prescribe. These skills depend on use of a knowledge base accumulated from experience, reading and previous teaching. If it were possible for computer-based diagnostic systems to provide diagnostic suggestions as accurately or (upsettingly) more accurately than dermatologists, one significant and fundamental part of the dermatologist's professional status would be eroded. If, or when, this happens it will indeed be necessary to readjust the role of a dermatologist; this role realignment will also be necessary when effective patient-individualized management advice systems become available. Computer-aided diagnosis or management systems will therefore pose a major challenge to professional status; dermatology as a speciality is, however, more likely to be successful if it embraces and encourages these new techniques than if it discourages them, thereby allowing non-dermatologists to take the lead in this area.

There are two major philosophical approaches to the problem of computer diagnosis. The first is a statistical epidemiological approach, and the second is a knowledge-based approach dependent on using 'experience' from practising clinicians. The statistical approach is scientifically and mathematically 'sounder', whereas the knowledge-based approach may be more applicable to dermatology, where statistics and epidemiological data on less common diseases are hard to come by.

In the statistical approach, very large numbers of patients with a particular disease need to be examined and the incidence of signs and symptoms in that disease determined. At the same time the incidence of the disease in the community and the incidence of the same symptoms and signs occurring in the general 'fit' population need to be determined. Armed with this information, it is possible using Bayes' theorem to give values to how much the presence or absence of a symptom or sign contributes to a change in likelihood of a disease being present. The more pieces of relevant information that are known about, the more accurate will be the resulting disease likelihood.

This approach to medical computer diagnosis has been widely used in other fields of medicine, such as classically in the diagnosis of abdominal pain, and in dermatology in the diagnosis of polymyositis and dermatomyositis[15]. In this paper[15] 153 patients were analysed, an indication of the large amount of statistical information needed to create a useful database. Ashton, Brooks and Pethybridge (personal communication) are undertaking a much larger survey of patients attending a dermatology clinic; several thousand patients had been documented in a standard detailed fashion by 1987 in an attempt to provide a much firmer basis for determining disease probability.

This approach is philosophically satisfying and appropriate for documentation of common diseases. Unfortunately, it becomes less helpful for very rare conditions, where the prior probability of a disease occurring in the population under study is extremely low.

The alternative approach to computer diagnosis is therefore quite different in concept. In the use of 'expert systems', the knowledge of an expert or of experts is distilled into a series of rules that encapsulate the main thought processes used when making particular diagnoses. The rules are eventually used to reach a diagnosis in response to information given about a particular patient.

These rules describe how an 'expert' thinks, and are each simple statements, unremarkable in themselves, exactly parallel in concept to 'rules of thumb' or 'classical signs' or simple descriptions used when teaching dermatology to medical students. There needs, however, to be a very large number of rules to describe even a simple diagnostic decision, and the extracting of these rules is a challenging and informative process, often making the 'expert' only too aware of how his thought processes are in fact 'inexpert' and non-logical.

Once the expert's knowledge is encapsulated in a series of rules, the knowledge is accessed in the program in a non-sequential manner so that appropriate questions can be posed and responses given by the computer program to the system user needing advice. When the system is in use, it is possible for the user to review the logical steps based on rules that the program has taken in order to reach that point. This ability to review the workings of the program is in contrast to the inability of a user to probe a statistically based program, where the calculations are often difficult to comprehend.

Whereas the statistically based diagnostic program needs to be based on published figures of symptom incidence and disease frequency, the expert system is based on an individual's uncheckable and arbitrary opinion. These concepts of information transmission are acceptable to most doctors; we are after all totally familiar with the concept of signed articles and accept that the information given reflects the opinion of the stated author. Expert systems therefore, can also be 'signed', in that those people who have created the rules can be identified.

In a rule-based knowledge system, it is possible to give useful and detailed diagnostic information about very rare diseases on which there is either little statistical information, or for which the very low incidence would always swamp the likelihood of a diagnosis being made. Expert systems, in contrast, are well suited for example to giving diagnostic advice on the ichthyoses[16].

The future potential for the application of expert systems in dermatology is immense[17]. Haberman *et al.*[18] in Toronto have described DIAG, an expert-system-based diagnostic program that has been under clinical trial and continual modification since 1982. Although its accuracy is often very good, full clinical acceptance has not yet been achieved.

It is easy to become overenthusiastic about the potential advantages that computer technology will confer on the practice of dermatology: do we in fact need help with diagnosis? Although most dermatological diagnosis is clinically straightforward, we all at times seek advice and help either from colleagues with a special interest or from the major textbooks: it is as an adjunct to this situation that computer diagnostic advice may be helpful to dermatologists. The potential advantages to doctors without dermatological training may be greater, where the frequency of need for advice may be higher. This leads to the next subject.

## TEACHING

There is a major need for more effective ways of teaching clinical dermatology. In the United Kingdom, for example, where there are only 230 dermatologists serving a population of 55 million on a referral basis, most skin problems are dealt with by general practitioners, who may have had only a minimal undergraduate dermatology training and little or no formal postgraduate dermatology training.

Even in those Western countries with direct primary patient access to dermatologists where the numbers of specialists are much greater, the extremely high incidence of skin disease in the community still inevitably results in many minor disorders being dealt with by non-dermatologists. In complete contrast, in many Third World countries the number of doctors with dermatology expertise is grossly inadequate. It is apparent, therefore, that attempts must be made to improve both availability and techniques of teaching dermatology.

Perhaps the most effective method of teaching clinical dermatology is by the apprentice system, where a doctor in training is attached to a department and through attending the clinics and ward work with the dermatologists, gradually takes over more responsibilities under supervision. Formal tutorials, lectures and structured reading, preferably with the goal of passing a specialist dermatology examination, usefully supplement this. The major advantage of the apprentice system and small tutorial teaching is that the teaching is inter-active; there is a two-way flow between the teacher and student that is stimulating, encouraging and by its nature adjusts to the student's personal training needs or level of understanding. Lectures and videotapes have the advantage of presenting structured information, and as clinical dermatology is a very 'visual' subject, it may be illustrated well in this format: the problem with these methods is that the student is passive and does not need to interact with the teacher.

The advent of computer-based teaching brings the potential to transform teaching programmes, by combining the advantages of several established teaching techniques. The most important inherent advantage of computer-assisted learning (or CAL) is that it is inter-active[19]. It does not, however, have the disadvantages of communication with a human being who tires, and who needs to be paid, usually on a time basis rather than on the basis of successful teaching: the computer program is infinitely patient. A second major advantage of CAL in dermatology is that, with the use of video disks, high-quality visual material can be accessed instantly, so that visual information can be presented flexibly as a response to a student's queries, rather than in a fixed sequence as in a lecture or on a teaching slide programme. Finally, once the teaching program is written, it can of course be used anywhere a suitable computer is available.

The use of a computer model for teaching in dermatology was first described by Short and Hess[20], and over the last few years further more sophisticated programs have been written. The effort needed to write an effective teaching program is considerable. At the present time, despite the clear massive worldwide potential need for suitable teaching material, the present market potential is not yet perceived as sufficiently strong for many centres to be investing in producing teaching programs. As the exponential growth rate in computer availability continues, this market situation is likely to change, and the demand for computer teaching programs to increase dramatically.

A number of pharmaceutical companies both in the UK and in the USA have produced CAL programs for teaching about specific areas, usually in relation to particular products. These have been effective teaching tools and have been popular when on display at dermatology meetings. It is, of course, possible to assess more objectively the success of such programs by incorporating pre- and post-testing of knowledge.

Simpson has described how (anonymous) information from the use of teaching programs can be used to assess the state of knowledge of a group of dermatologists: such techniques could be used to identify deficiencies in training or areas where specific postgraduate training should be targeted.

## RESEARCH

It is unlikely that there is anyone involved in dermatology research who does not use a computer in the work. The ability of computer programs to handle and manipulate large amounts of data easily make their use almost essential for the day-to-day handling of information gained from both laboratory-based and clinical research work. A large number of computer programs are available for the statistical analysis of information gained in studies, and the availability of these within a department has transformed the ease with which statistical comparisons can be made. The general use of data storage and analysis in dermatology research is universally beneficial.

An example of a recent positive use of computer analysis of a large group of patients in a clinical study is given by Jeanmougin and Civatte[21]. In a multicentre study, 193 patients with photodermatoses were studied, and computer analysis revealed amongst these patients a new entity now termed 'benign summer light eruption'.

In a wider context, the use of computers is central in major epidemiological studies designed to give information on risk factors in skin disease. In Sweden, a country where a unique personal identifying number is used for many different records, it has been possible to gain very complete information using data linkage between treatment records and a cancer registry. This study[22] provided evidence that the risk of malignant skin tumours after grenz-ray treatment for benign skin tumours is small. It was computer-based population patient information that made this study possible, a technique which, incidentally, caused some controversy in another study when the subject under review was the relationship of abortion to cancer later in life.

There are, of course, a large number of specific research techniques and instrumentations in dermatology that rely on computer interaction. It is impossible to list all of these, but there are three techniques currently in use in the dermatology department in Cardiff that illustrate the diverse ways in which computer technology can contribute to our understanding of the skin.

## Image analysis

Both the clinical practice of dermatology and the inherently integrated service of dermatopathology rely heavily on the interpretation of visual information by clinician and pathologist. Although the human eye and brain are excellent at pattern recognition and at assessing comparisons between visual patterns when presented together, our ability to assign consistent quantification to size, pattern or colour from week to week is poor. In daily clinical practice this is not a major handicap, as we are used to dealing in a clinical world of inexact recording of clinical status; it would none the less be highly desirable to record objectively the severity of our patient's disease. In research work, the difficulties posed by our variable subjective recording of, say, psoriatic plaque area or epidermal cell size result in much greater problems. It is for these reasons that computer-based image analysis techniques are being applied to dermatology.

Using an image analysis computer, a black and white video image of a histological slide, or of a photograph, or directly of a patient is analysed in terms of degrees of density at each point on the image. By altering the 'cut-off' point of the grey level required, it is possible to highlight areas on the image of the same degree of greyness or within the same range of greyness. Once an area is thus identified, it is possible to instantly measure its area and, for example, compare one highlighted area with another. In addition, using a light pen, other areas on the screen can be identified and similar calculations may take place with reference to that newly defined site. It is possible to imagine how this technique could be used to measure a patient's area of psoriasis involvement[23] or, on histology slides, areas or numbers of nuclei. The technique may also be used to assess objectively skin surface texture[24]. There are a number of difficulties with this method: in particular, the levels of greyness corresponding to identical features may differ because of lighting or differing angles of the lesion on a curved body surface. The concept does, however, work in many applications and signposts the way to more objective scientific methodology for recording skin disease.

A clever application of the vast information-managing power of computers is the ability to reconstruct three-dimensional images from two-dimensional data. Lea *et al.*[25] have described how ultrathin serial sections of naevi and the basement membrane zone can be used to create such information. Similarly, Gebhart *et al.*[26] have shown how estimates of malignant melanoma volumes can be made with computer assistance.

It is suggested by Cascinelli *et al.*[27] that image analysis techniques may be useful for diagnostic purposes. They describe the results of image analysis of colour slides of cutaneous melanoma, and suggest the possibility of similar analysis of histological sections simultaneously to gain additional information. The prospects for the use of this technique are indeed very exciting.

## HPLC analysis

The control and supervision of high-pressure liquid chromatography analysis is a time-consuming task often demanding repetitive work. In the Cardiff dermatology department, such instrumentation is used to measure drug levels in blood, urine, skin and other appendages. In the newer instrumentation now being used, the major control of the throughput of samples and controls is under the instruction of a computer, which also initially analyses the results and displays them graphically. This facility frees the technician for other tasks during a long run of sample analysis.

## Physical properties of nails

Another example of the frequent marrying of laboratory instruments and computers is given by the methods we are currently devising to measure the physical properties of nails. One of these instruments is designed to give an objective measure of the contour of nails (Finlay, Western, Edwards (unpublished)). Sensors that detect the nail contour send signals to a BBC B microcomputer, which, despite the age of its design, is still an excellent laboratory computer instrument. Objective measures of the nail contour are then recorded, analysed and displayed. Such instrumentation, although possible in theory to devise without computer analysis, would be clumsy and much more tedious to use without this support.

## CONCLUSION

### Cutaneous problems with computers

Although this article concerns the benefits of the application of computers to dermatological practice, it behoves the clinical dermatologist to be at least aware of the cutaneous problems that have been blamed on video display terminals. There have been several reports of facial rashes occurring in people working with computers, and these have been well reviewed by Berg and Liden[28]. One hypothesis is that electrostatic field charges cause a deposition of air pollutants on the skin, causing irritation or aggravating pre-existing skin disease. The frequency of these problems is extremely low, so the risk of developing this problem must not be used as an excuse by the keyboard-shy dermatologist to remain a computer novice.

Even given the many advantages of using a computer in a hospital- or office-based dermatology department, some may still be unconvinced. Rigel[29] gives some guidance for the doubters, but surely a dermatology practice without the advantages of computer facilities will soon be viewed as eccentric. In the 1980s, when there is now even a microcomputer program to help us avoid sunburn[30], and 1990s, most aspects of our professional lives are likely to be influenced by computer technology.

### Contact for advice in the United Kingdom

The Chairman or Secretary, Computer Application Working Group, c/o British Association of Dermatologists, 6, St Andrew's Place, Regent's Park, London NW1 4LB.

## Recommended reading

Rigel, D.S. and Rosenthal L.E. (guest editors) (1986). Computers in dermatology. *Dermatol. Clin.*, **4**(4).

## REFERENCES


1. Shrank, A.B. (1987). *B.A.D. Looks at Word Processors.* (London: British Association of Dermatologists).
2. Henderson, A.S. *et al.* (1983). Computers in medicine. A simple system for references and reprints. *Br. Med. J.*, **287,** 1448–1449
3. Dyer, C. (1985). Data protection act and medical records. *Br. Med. J.*, **291,** 1070–1071
4. Macfarlane, H.A. *et al.* (1986). Use of a computer program for contact dermatitis clinic results. *Contact Dermatitis*, **14,** 162–4
5. Dooms-Goosens, A., Dooms, M., Drieghe, J. and Degreef, H. (1987). Computers and contact dermatitis. *Computer Workshop, XVII Congressus Mundi Dermatologiae (CMD), Volume of Abstracts Part 1*, p. 273. (Free University of Berlin)
6. Simpson, N.B., Kenny, G.N.C. and MacKenzie, J.A.B. (1986). Microcomputer management of chemotherapy for psoriasis. *Clin. Exp. Dermatol.*, **11,** 619–623
7. Torrence, I., Marks, J. and Canning, B. (1987). Use of a microcomputer to store and process clinical records in a Puva unit. *Computer Workshop, XVII Congressus Mundi Dermatologicae (CMD), Volume of Abstracts Part 1,* p. 274. (Free University of Berlin)
8. Alexander, S. and Shrank, A.B. (1978). *International Coding Index for Dermatology.* (Oxford: Blackwell Scientific)
9. White, R. (1986). Data base management systems. How they work in dermatology. *Dermatol. Clin.*, **4,** 569–578
10. Schoolman, H.M. (1986). The physician and the medical literature. From Index Medicus to MEDLARS to GRATEFUL MED and beyond. *Arch. Dermatol.*, **122,** 875–876
11. Rigel, D.S. (1987). Computers in dermatology. Review of communication software for dermatology. *J. Am. Acad. Dermatol.*, **16,** 606–609
12. Kopf, A.W., Geronemus, R., Sanchez, M., Natow, A., Grossman, D. and Goldberg, D. (1986). DERM/RX: A computer aid to the management of diseases of the skin. *Dermatol. Clin.*, **4,** 589–598
13. Maddin, S. and Stern, R.S. (1986). DERM/PHARM: Drug data base for dermatologists. *Dermatol. Clin.*, **4,** 599–606
14. Norins, A.L. (1964). Computers in dermatology. *Arch. Dermatol.*, **90,** 506–511
15. Bohan, A., Peter, J.B., Bowman, R.L. and Pearson, C.M. (1977). A computer-assisted analysis of 153 patients with polymyositis and dermatomyositis. *Medicine*, **56,** 255–286
16. Finlay, A.Y., Sinclair, J. and Alty, J.L. (1987). Expert system diagnosis of ichthyosis. *Clin. Exp. Dermatol.*, **12,** 239–240
17. Finlay, A.Y. and Hammond, P. (1986). Expert systems in dermatology: the computer potential. The example of facial tumour diagnosis. *Dermatologica*, **173,** 79–84

18. Haberman, H.F., Norwich, K.H., Diehl, D.L., Evans, S.J., Harvey, B., Landau, J., Cobbold, R.S.C., O'Beirne, H. and Zingg, W. (1985). DIAG: A computer-assisted dermatologic diagnostic system – clinical experience and insight. *J. Am. Acad. Dermatol.*, **12,** 132–143
19. Simpson, N.B. (1987). CAL for Undergraduates. *Computer Workshop, XVII Congressus Mundi Dermatologiae (CMD), Volume of Abstracts Part 1*, pp. 274–275. (Free University of Berlin)
20. Short, J.M. and Hess, A.C. (1980). Simulation of skin diseases for teaching dermatological diagnoses. *J. Med. Educ.*, **55,** 377
21. Jeanmougin, M. and Civatte, J. (1986) Benign summer light eruption: a new entity? *Arch. Dermatol.*, **122,** 376
22. Lindelof, B. and Eklund, G. (1986). Incidence of malignant skin tumours in 14,140 patients after grenz-ray treatment for benign skin disorders. *Arch. Dermatol.*, **122,** 1391–1395
23. Marks, R., Barton, S.P., Shuttleworth, D. and Finlay, A.Y. (1988). Assessment of disease progress in psoriasis. *Arch. Dermatol.* (in press)
24. Barton, S.P., Marshall, R.J. and Marks, R. (1987). A novel method for assessing skin surface topography. *Bioeng. Skin*, **3,** 93–107
25. Lea, P.J. *et al.* (1986). Human melanocytic naevi. 1. Electron microscopy and 3-dimensional reconstruction of naevi and basement membrane zone from ultrathin serial sections. *Acta. Derm. Venereol. (Stockh.) Suppl.*, **127,** 5–15
26. Gebhart, W. *et al.* (1984). Computer assisted volumetric analysis of cutaneous malignant melanomas. *Am. J. Dermatopathol. Suppl.*, **6,** 93–95
27. Cascinelli, N., Ferrario, M., Tonelli, T. and Leo, E. (1987). A possible new tool for clinical diagnosis of melanoma: The computer. *J. Am. Acad. Dermatol.*, **16,** 361–367
28. Berg, M. and Liden, S. (1987). Skin problems in video display terminal users. *J. Am. Acad. Dermatol.*, **17,** 682–683
29. Rigel, D.S. (1985). Is it time for a computer in your practice? V. How to evaluate if a computer is appropriate for your practice. *J. Dermatol. Surg. Oncol.*, **11,** 215–216
30. Diffey, B. (1984). Using a microcomputer program to avoid sunburn. *Photodermatology*, **1,** 45–51

# INDEX